Frontiers in Clinical Drug Research - CNS and Neurological Disorders

(Volume 8)

Edited by

Atta-ur-Rahman, *FRS*

Kings College
University of Cambridge, Cambridge
UK

&

Zareen Amtul

The University of Windsor
Department of Chemistry and Biochemistry
Windsor, ON
Canada

Frontiers in Clinical Drug Research - CNS and Neurological Disorders

Volume # 8

Editors: Atta-ur-Rahman, *FRS* and Zareen Amtul

ISSN (Online): 2214-7527

ISSN (Print): 2451-8883

ISBN (Online): 978-981-14-7008-0

ISBN (Print): 978-981-14-7006-6

ISBN (Paperback): 978-981-14-7007-3

need for a court order if at any point you breach any terms of this License Agreement. In no event will any delay or failure by Bentham Science Publishers in enforcing your compliance with this License Agreement constitute a waiver of any of its rights.

3. You acknowledge that you have read this License Agreement, and agree to be bound by its terms and conditions. To the extent that any other terms and conditions presented on any website of Bentham Science Publishers conflict with, or are inconsistent with, the terms and conditions set out in this License Agreement, you acknowledge that the terms and conditions set out in this License Agreement shall prevail.

Bentham Science Publishers Pte. Ltd.
80 Robinson Road #02-00
Singapore 068898
Singapore
Email: subscriptions@benthamscience.net

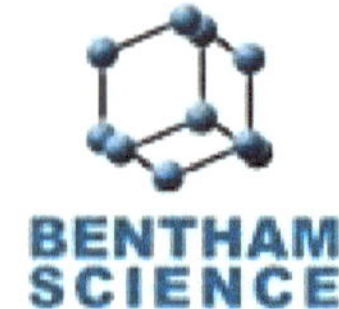

CONTENTS

PREFACE

Neurodegenerative disorders are some of the overwhelming challenges modern medicine is facing. To find efficacious treatments for these disorders, we still need to advance our understanding of the various events and cellular processes that lead to neurodegeneration. These include pathological protein aggregation and factors that cause the death of neuronal cells.

Volume 8 of our book series *Frontiers in Clinical Drug Research - CNS and Neurological Disorders* features a set of exciting and remarkable new research projects presented by an emerging and expert panel of researchers. They have reviewed innovative research studies that could lead to a richer interpretation of the essentials needed to understand the nerve cell functions and/or failures.

This book presents cutting-edge, and in-depth investigations that outline neurodegeneration at the cellular level. It discusses new trends in neurodegenerative research aimed to slow down the progression of neurological ailments, offering hope to people with these debilitating and at times incurable illness. Thus chapter 1 covers the current knowledge and perspectives surrounding the emerging innovative therapies of spinal muscular atrophy, as well as pin-pointing the molecules that offer potential new treatments for this debilitating condition. Chapter 2 highlights the obesity induced by the usage of neurological drugs such as antiepileptic, antipsychotic, and antidepressant drugs. Chapter 3 discusses the development of new therapeutic targets based on the understanding of the molecular mechanisms that lead to infectious, functional, structural, and degenerative disorders of the nervous system. Chapter 4 briefly reviews the screening models for neuroleptic drug-induced hyperprolactinemia. The last chapter 5 evaluates the glioma imaging modalities and the novel agents that are being implicated to image glioma.

In short, this book presents a scholarly collection of research articles from the budding as well as established scientists in the field. It is hoped that the presentations will lead to a better understanding by the neuroscience community of the underlying mechanisms of brain disorders, leading to more effective treatments.

We are grateful for the timely efforts made by the editorial personnel, especially Mr. Mahmood Alam (Director Publications), and Mrs. Salma Sarfaraz (Senior Manager Publications) at Bentham Science Publishers.

Atta-ur-Rahman, *FRS*
Honorary Life Fellow
Kings College
University of Cambridge
Cambridge
UK

Zareen Amtul
The University of Windsor
Department of Chemistry and Biochemistry
Windsor, ON
Canada

List of Contributors

Betul Cevik	Tokat Gaziosmanpasa University, Faculty of Medicine, Department of Neurology, Tokat, Turkey
Ching H. Wang	Department of Neurology, Driscoll Children's Hospital, Corpus Christi, Texas, USA College of Medicine, Texas A&M University, College Station, Texas, USA
Durdane Aksoy	Tokat Gaziosmanpasa University, Faculty of Medicine, Department of Neurology, Tokat, Turkey
Farhin Patel	Department of Biological Sciences, P. D. Patel Institute of Applied Sciences, Charotar Universityof Science and Technology, Changa, Anand- 388421, Gujarat, India
Mine Silindir-Gunay	Hacettepe University, Faculty of Pharmacy, Department of Radiopharmacy, 06100, Sıhhiye, Ankara, Turkey
Orhan Sumbul	Tokat Gaziosmanpasa University, Faculty of Medicine, Department of Neurology, Tokat, Turkey
Palash Mandal	Department of Biological Sciences, P. D. Patel Institute of Applied Sciences, Charotar University of Science and Technology, Changa, Anand- 388421, Gujarat, India
Prashant Tiwari	School of Pharmacy, School of Health and Allied Sciences, ARKA JAIN University, Jamshedpur -832102, India
Pratap Kumar Sahu	Department of Pharmacology, School of Pharmaceutical Sciences, Siksha O Anusandhan (Deemed to be University), Bhubaneswar - 751029, India
Semiha Kurt	Tokat Gaziosmanpasa University, Faculty of Medicine, Department of Neurology, Tokat, Turkey
Shweta Shrivastava	School of Pharmacy, School of Health and Allied Sciences, ARKA JAIN University, Jamshedpur -832102, India
Sunil Kumar Dubey	Institute of Pharmacy, Birla Institute of Technology and Science, Pilani, Rajasthan - 333031, India
Tai-Heng Chen	Section of Neurobiology, Department of Biological Sciences, University of Southern California, Los Angeles, California, USA Department of Pediatrics, Kaohsiung Medical University Hospital, Kaohsiung Medical University, Kaohsiung, Taiwan School of Post-Baccalaureate Medicine, College of Medicine, Kaohsiung Medical University, Kaohsiung, Taiwan

CHAPTER 1

Emerging Innovative Therapies of Spinal Muscular Atrophy: Current Knowledge and Perspectives

Tai-Heng Chen[1,2,3,*] and **Ching H. Wang**[4,5]

[1] *Section of Neurobiology, Department of Biological Sciences, University of Southern California, Los Angeles, California, USA*

[2] *Department of Pediatrics, Kaohsiung Medical University Hospital, Kaohsiung Medical University, Kaohsiung, Taiwan*

[3] *School of Post-Baccalaureate Medicine, College of Medicine, Kaohsiung Medical University, Kaohsiung, Taiwan*

[4] *Department of Neurology, Driscoll Children's Hospital, Corpus Christi, Texas, USA*

[5] *College of Medicine, Texas A&M University, College Station, Texas, USA*

Abstract: Spinal muscular atrophy (SMA) is a rare neuromuscular disorder characterized by the degeneration of motor neurons (MNs) in the spinal cord resulting in progressive muscle atrophy and weakness. Due to its early onset and severity of symptoms, SMA is notable in the health care community as one of the most common causes of early infant death. SMA is caused by missing a functional survival motor neuron 1 (*SMN1*) gene in patients who produce deficient levels of survival motor neuron (SMN) protein from a copy gene (*SMN2*), but that could not sustain the survival of spinal cord MNs. Before the end of 2016, there was no cure for SMA, and management only consisted of supportive care. Since then, several therapeutic strategies to increase SMN protein have developed and are currently in various stages of clinical trials. The *SMN2*-directed antisense oligonucleotide (ASO) therapy was first approved by the FDA in December 2017. Subsequently, in May 2019, gene therapy using an adeno-associated viral vector to deliver the DNA sequence of SMN protein was also approved. These two novel therapeutics have a common objective: to increase the production of SMN protein in MNs, and thereby improve motor function and survival. Treating patients with SMA brings new responsibilities and unique dilemmas. As SMA is such a devastating disease, it is reasonable to assume that a single therapeutic modality may not be sufficient. Neither therapy currently available provides a complete cure. Several other treatment strategies are currently under investigation. These include: establishing an early diagnosis to enable early treatment, a combination of the different treatment regimens, and frequency, dosage, and route variations of drug delivery. Understanding the underlying mechanisms of these treatments is the other area of needed study.

---

* **Corresponding author Dr. Tai-Heng Chen:** Kaohsiung Medical University Hospital No. 100, Tzyou 1st Road, Kaohsiung 80708, Taiwan; Tel: +886-7-312-1101 ; Fax: +886-7-321-2062; E-mail address: taihen@kmu.edu.tw

Keywords: Clinical trial, Novel therapy, Spinal muscular atrophy, Survival motor neuron protein.

INTRODUCTION

Spinal muscular atrophy (SMA) is an autosomal recessive neuromuscular disorder caused by the degeneration of alpha motor neurons (MNs) in the spinal cord leading to muscle atrophy and weakness. Although recognized as a rare disease with an estimated worldwide incidence of ~1/10,000 live births, SMA is the second most common autosomal recessive genetic disorder and the most common monogenic disease-causing early infant death [1, 2]. The carrier frequency varies from 1 in 38 to 1 in 72, among different ethnic groups with a pan-ethnic average of 1/54 [3].

SMA was firstly reported in two infant brothers by Guido Werdnig in 1891 and later seven additional patients by Johan Hoffmann from 1893 to 1900 [4]. In 1995, scientists discovered the genetic basis of SMA, which involved the missing of a functional survival motor neuron 1 (*SMN1*) gene [5]. About 95% of SMA cases are caused by mutations or deletions in the *SMN1* gene in chromosome 5q11.2–q13.3.2, thus termed as 5q SMA. Deletion or mutation of the *SMN1* gene results in lacking the production of survival motor neuron (SMN) protein, a vital protein that enables the survival of spinal cord MNs. The degeneration of MNs, in turn, causes widespread muscle atrophy and weakness, the primary symptoms of SMA [3, 6].

At the molecular level, SMN protein acts as a multifunctional protein ubiquitously expressed in almost all somatic cells. SMN is involved in many cellular functions, including mRNA editing, splicing, and axonal transport [7]. The most appreciated canonical role of SMN is to serve as an essential ribonucleoprotein (RNP) for mRNA splicing. SMN protein is embedded in a complex with seven Gemins and UNR-interacting protein (UNRIP) that shuttles Sm protein onto nascent uridine-rich noncoding RNAs (snRNAs) upon their export to the cytoplasm, thereby creating small nuclear RNPs (snRNPs) that form spliceosomes in the nucleus [8 - 10]. In addition to facilitating snRNP assembly, the SMN complex plays a role in assisting arginine methylation of specific splicing-related proteins that are involved in pre-mRNA splicing [11, 12]. All cells are dependent upon SMN, but the reduction in snRNPs assembly can be particularly critical for specific cell types, particularly in MNs. Studies on SMA animal models have revealed a direct correlation between the ability to assemble snRNPs and SMA severity, and delivery of mature snRNPs even without the SMN component is sufficient to rescue SMA phenotypes [13 - 15]. Such an outcome implies that SMN protein levels might affect the splicing of SMN pre-mRNA to include exon 7 through an autoregulatory loop, thereby influencing a general process of snRNP biogenesis [16]. Besides the canonical role of SMN in the splicing machinery, other studies have highlighted its multiple roles in cellular functions. For example, the recruitment of SMN protein is also involved in many other essential cellular pathways, including DNA repair and protein and mRNA transportation along axons of MNs [17 - 19]. Collectively, studies to date support that loss of SMN-RNP complex assembly and its activity results in a series of different cellular pathways that lead to SMA. However, it is still unclear how a deficiency in the ubiquitously expressed SMN protein can selectively cause the degeneration of MNs [7]. Increasing evidence suggests SMN playing a pivotal role beyond the MNs. The autoregulatory mechanism of SMN may explain the more detrimental effects of SMN deficiency that could result in the selective MN degeneration in SMA. Nevertheless, the multifaceted roles of SMN protein are still under investigation, and it is unclear how a deficiency in ubiquitously expressed SMN can selectively cause the dramatic MN degeneration. The cell autonomous effects related to deficient SMN are responsible for the MNs degeneration; however, it does not account for the full SMA phenotype, implicating not only dysfunction of neural networks but other non-neuronal cell types involved in the disease process [20, 21]. For example, recent studies point that the MN survival and functionality of SMA animal and cellular models are highly dependent on glial cells, which play an essential role in neuronal communication and neuroinflammation [22, 23]. These findings imply that SMA could also be a neuroinflammatory disease.

Fig. (**1**) illustrates the genetic basis and pathogenesis of SMA. It also explains the cause of phenotypic variations. Complete loss of SMN protein resulted from deletion/mutations of *smn* or *SMN1* (in humans and bonobos only) leads to embryonic lethality to all species [24, 25]. In the genomes of higher primate species, including humans, there is a nearly identical copy of *SMN1*, called *SMN2* [5]. *SMN2* differs from *SMN1* by a single nucleotide (C-to-T) substitution in the exon 7. This single base-pair variation leads to skipping of exon 7 during RNA splicing and produces an *SMN2* transcript lacking exon 7, called SMNΔ7. Unlike the *SMN1* gene, only a small amount of full-length (FL) mRNA is produced by the *SMN2* gene due to this skipping of exon 7 during RNA splicing [26]. In contrast to the FL-SMN protein, SMN generated by the SMNΔ7 transcript cannot oligomerize efficiently, resulting in truncated morphology, which is degraded rapidly [7, 9]. In SMA patients, alternative splicing in the *SMN2* gene allows it to produce only ~10% of FL-SMN transcripts and protein. This low amount of SMN protein is sufficient to prevent embryonic lethality, but cannot fully compensate for the missing *SMN1*. In the human genome, there are variable numbers of *SMN2* gene copies, and the amount of SMN protein produced is directly correlated with the copy number of the *SMN2* gene. Consequently, the SMA severity is inversely related to the number of the *SMN2* gene copy; the higher the copy number, the less severe the SMA phenotype. However, this phenotype-genotype correlation can be affected by other factors. Recent studies showed that other cellular mechanisms, like positive or negative disease modifiers, may also involve in the modulation of SMA clinical severity. For example, rare *SMN2* variants (c.859G>C), as well as independent modifiers such as plastin 3 or neurocalcin delta, can further influence the disease severity [27 - 29]. In brief, the loss of the *SMN1* gene leads to SMA, whose severity is partially modified by various copies of *SMN2*.

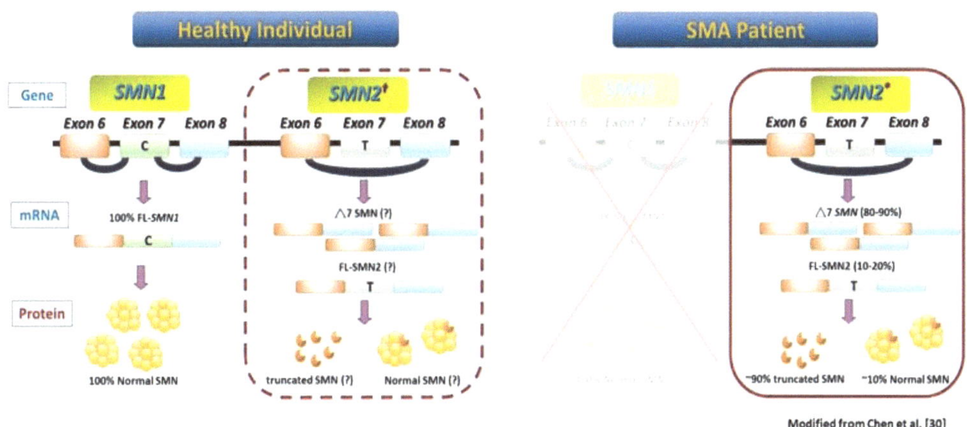

Fig. (1).   Genetic basis of spinal muscular atrophy (SMA) [30]. In a healthy individual, full-length (FL) survival motor neuron (SMN) mRNA and protein arise from the *SMN1* gene. Patients with SMA have homozygous deletion or mutation of *SMN1* but retain at least one *SMN2* (indicated with an asterisk in the solid-border box on the right). However, *SMN2* can be dispensable in a healthy individual (indicated with an obelisk in the dotted-border box on the left). This single-nucleotide change in exon 7 (C-to-T) of *SMN2* causes alternative splicing during transcription, resulting in most *SMN2* mRNA lacking exon 7 (Δ7 SMN). About 90% of Δ7 SMN transcripts produce unstable truncated SMN protein, but a minority include exon 7 and code for FL, which maintains a degree of MN survival.

CLINICAL CHARACTERISTICS OF SMA

The most severe type of SMA presents in infancy. Correlated with the onset of symptoms, here is a rapid and catastrophic loss of connectivity between MNs and their innervated muscles with depletion of neuronal endplates [1, 3]. As a consequence of MN degeneration, progressive muscle wasting and weakness become the main feature of SMA. These clinical symptoms presented with a spectrum of severity ranging from extremely compromised neonates with immediate respiratory failure to late-onset, minimal limb weakness in adulthood. However, unlike the relentless decline of motor function observed in other motor neuron disease (MND) like amyotrophic lateral sclerosis, patients with intermediate and milder forms of SMA tend to maintain their level of motor function over many years [31 - 33]. Interestingly, cognitive function is generally intact in patients with SMA, and they often have higher than average intelligence [1].

Phenotypes and Classifications of SMA

SMA presents with a broad range of clinical severity, such as the age of onset and rate of progression. There are variabilities between and within each phenotypic subtype that constitutes a clinical continuum [34, 35] In general, SMA is classified into three main phenotypes based on age at symptoms/signs onset, and highest motor function achieved [3, 29, 35]. However, some patients with SMA are outliers on either end of the phenotypic spectrum. Besides, subclassification has also been proposed in SMA types 1 and 3, and sometimes in type 2 phenotype Table **1**.

At the most severe end of the spectrum, patients with type 0 SMA (categorized into type 1A by some authors) are usually associated with prenatal onset of signs, such as a history of decreased fetal movements [36]. These rare cases usually present with arthrogryposis multiplex congenital and have profound hypotonia and respiratory distress soon after birth [37]. Life expectancy is extremely short, and if untreated, most of them are unable to survive beyond one month of age [1, 38].

Table 1. Classification and subtypes of spinal muscular atrophy.

SMA Type (Historical name)	OMIM	Onset Age	Motor Milestones Achieved	Subclassfication	Natural History	Other Features	Estimated *SMN2* Copies	Estimated SMA Proportion
Type 0	-	Prenatal or at birth	Never sits Never head control	-	Death < 1 mo if untreated	Joint contractures, cardiac defect; facial diplegia; immediate respiratory failure after birth	1 *SMN2* copy in ~100% of patients	Unclear, Maybe <1%
Type 1 (Werdnig-Hoffmann disease)	253300	0–6 mo	Never sits, some achieve head control	1A: onset <1 mo, usually by 2 wk; absent head control 1B: onset 1-3 mo; poor or absent head control 1C: onset 3-6 mo, head control achieved	1A: death <6 mo if untreated 1B and 1C: death <2 yr if untreated	1A: very similar to type 0 SMA 1B and 1C: tongue fasciculation; swallowing difficulties; early respiratory failure	1 or 2 *SMN2* Copies in ~80% of patients	~60%

(Table 1) cont.....

SMA Type (Historical name)	OMIM	Onset Age	Motor Milestones Achieved	Subclassfication	Natural History	Other Features	Estimated *SMN2* Copies	Estimated SMA Proportion
Type 2 (Dubowitz disease)	253550	7–18 mo	Sits but never stands	2A: Sits independently, may loses the ability to sit in later life 2B: Sits independently, Maintains the ability to sit * According to functional level, decimal classification ranging from 2.1 to 2.9	Usually survive >2 yr ; ~70% alive at 25 yr	Proximal weakness; postural hand tremor; normal intellectual ability; kyphoscoliosis	3 *SMN2* copies in >70% patients	~27%
Type 3 (Kugelberg-Welander disease)	253400	>18 mo	Stands and walks	3A: onset between 18 and 36 mo 3B: onset >3 yr	Survival into adulthood	May have hand tremor; resembles muscular dystrophy 3A: Scoliosis; usually early loss of ambulation	3 or 4 *SMN2* copies in ~95% of patients	~12%
Type 4	271150	10–30 yr, usually >21 yr	Stands and walks	-	Survival into adulthood	Usually preserved walking ability	4 or more *SMN2* copies in >90%	~1%

SMA: spinal muscular atrophy; mo: months; yr: years

Type 1 SMA patients account for more than 50% of the total incidence of SMA. As a general rule, infants with *SMN1* biallelic deletions and only two copies of *SMN2* have a 97% risk of this most severe phenotype of SMA. These patients usually present with symptoms onset before six months and are described as non-sitters because they never achieve independent sitting, which is the beginning of all major motor milestones. Notably, congenital heart defect is a feature of severe SMA phenotype, especially in SMA types 0 and 1 [39]. Respiratory muscle dysfunction attributes to most cases of mortality within the first two years of life. Studies of SMA natural history showed the median age of death is 13.5 months and the need for permanent ventilation (>16 hours per day) at 10.5 months for patients with two copies of *SMN2* [40, 41].

Patients with the intermediate severity of type 2 SMA (Dubowitz's disease) usually develop weakness within 7–18 months of age. Failure to achieve the major developmental milestones of independent walking brought these patients to clinical attention. Patients usually exhibit areflexia and proximal weakness that is more severe in the lower extremities than upper extremities. Although these patients can maintain a sitting position unaided (thus named "sitters") and some can even stand with leg braces, none can walk independently. Fine tremors with digit extension or hand grips are commonly observed. Due to the wide variation of symptom severities in this group of patients, further classification has been proposed to subdivide them into 2.1 to 2.9 subtypes within type 2 SMA based on their functional levels [38, 42]. Weak swallowing might deter weight gain. Kyphoscoliosis usually develops and can result in a restrictive lung disease if not intervened by surgical or orthotic procedures. Similar to patients with type 1 SMA, clearing of airway secretions and coughing becomes difficult because of poor bulbar function and weak intercostal muscles. The majority of patients with type 2 SMA can survive into adulthood, with 93% surviving to 25 years. However, these patients usually require aggressive supportive care due to compromised swallowing ability and respiratory issues when they enter the adolescent years [43].

Type 3 SMA is the mildest form of SMA (also called Kugelberg-Welander disease). Patients usually have symptoms onset around 1.5 years of age. They can stand unsupported and walk independently. However, these patients exhibit an extensive symptom heterogeneity and are sometimes misdiagnosed with myopathy or muscular dystrophy. These patients can be further divided into two subgroups according to their age of onset: patients with type 3A have an onset of symptoms between 18 months and three years, and patients with type 3B usually present after three years [32]. Their distribution of weakness is similar to that seen in patients with types 1 and 2 SMA, albeit of a much slower progression. Some patients may be ambulatory until their middle age [42]. In clinical trials, type 3 patients who lost their ability to walk independently in childhood are often grouped with the non-ambulatory patients, or sitters, because they can be assessed with the same outcome measures.

At the other mildest end of the spectrum is an adult-onset form, known as type 4 SMA, who presents onset symptoms, usually a weakness of lower extremities, after the second decade. Type 4 patients have a good prognosis with ambulation into adulthood and a mostly average life span [44].

The Implication of Phenotypic Classification in SMA Clinical Trials

Previous investigations concentrated on the natural history of SMA, and the efforts to develop standardized tools of outcome measures have assisted in achieving clinical trial readiness in the field [45, 46]. Early clinical trials used *SMN2* copy numbers as a criterion for patient enrollment [47]. However, studies showed that while patients with a higher number of *SMN2* copies generally have a milder phenotype, this prediction is not always accurate [29]. Other prognostic factors, such as the age of onset of symptoms within each SMA subtypes, have been identified [38].

Although the assignment of trial groups according to SMA subtypes (*i.e.,* types 1, 2, and 3) has some clinical advantages, it is not always the best way to stratify patients. Within each SMA subtype, there could be the heterogeneity of phenotypes due to different stages of disease progression (*e.g.,* some type 3 patients are still ambulatory, and some have lost it). Therefore, using the current motor function level (such as ambulant status) may be more relevant to clinical trial design and outcome measures. Several clinical trials have been conducted by stratifying patients into non-sitter, sitter, and walker to achieve the uniformity of functional level and use of appropriate outcome measures [48]. This approach acknowledges the SMA phenotypes as a continuum and focuses on the current functional status and the therapy response.

Furthermore, pulmonary function assessment may better reflect disease state than muscle strength [49]. Nevertheless, repeat evaluations are imperative before assigning a patient to a specific SMA type. In particular of patients with SMA types 2 and 3, the onset, time course, and extent of MN loss has not been well established, yet are vital in determining whether there is a specific therapeutic window for these patients with milder phenotypes.

IMPACTS OF EVOLVING SUPPORTIVE CARE IN SMA THERA-PEUTIC ERA

The successful disease modification of the newly developed therapies have altered the SMA clinical landscape and raised the needs for new supportive care and treatment guidelines [48, 50]. The need for multidisciplinary care standard for SMA patients was evident for quite sometime before the establishment of the standard of care (SOC) recommendations. Clinical outcome of SMA patients varies greatly depending on their demographic locations and the care they received. In 2007 a Consensus Statement for Standard of Care in Spinal Muscular Atrophy was published by an international multidisciplinary team addressing the comprehensive care standard for patients with SMA [51]. With the advent of disease-modifying treatments, and updated two-part SOC document was published in 2018 [52, 53]. The multidisciplinary team, which includes medical specialists in neurology, pulmonology, acute care, nutrition support, gastroenterology, orthopedics, physical therapy/rehabilitation, and other medical subspecialties, should continue to provide comprehensive care as the patients undergo specific therapies Fig. (**2**). Implementation of comprehensive SOC also plays a vital role in drug development because it eliminates the variability of treatment outcomes due to variable care received. Therefore, standardized care must be implemented for all patients participating in clinical trials [35, 48]. As such, updated SOC guidelines for SMA will continue to be necessary as more therapeutic modalities become available, and the definition of care standard may be changed with time.

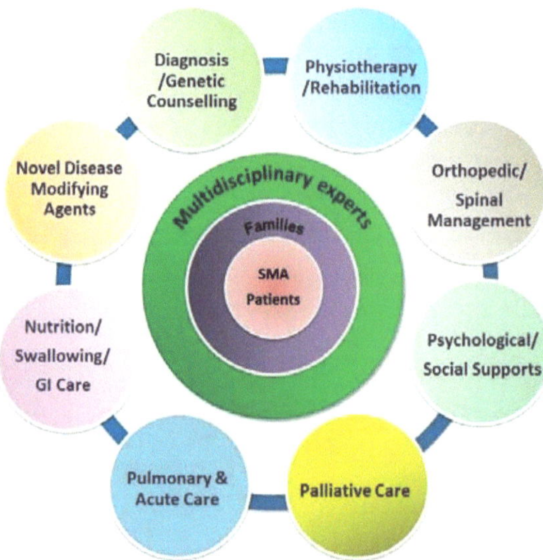

Fig. (2). Paradigm of multidisciplinary care of SMA, incorporating disease-modifying therapies with supportive care [30]. Novel disease-modifying medications and evolving multidisciplinary supportive management need to occur concomitantly to achieve the best possible outcome for SMA patients.

In the therapeutic era, we reasonably expect that type 1 SMA patients will likely transition into less severe types 3 and 4 once treated, giving them a more extended or average lifespan. It remains unclear whether persistent interventions will be required, and a complete long-term reversal of symptoms will be attained. Unfortunately, because there is a paucity of studies investigating the support and medical needs of type 4 SMA patients (and soon the treated patients), it is unknown whether such lifespan extension will reveal new, previously unknown, comorbidities that could arise with age in this new, modified SMA affected population. In parallel with pre-clinical advances, continued evolution in multidisciplinary care with technological advances should be pursued, particularly for those with milder phenotypes after disease-modifying therapy.

RECENT ADVANCES IN INNOVATIVE THERAPEUTICS IN SMA: FOCUSING ON SMN AND BEYOND

In general, the therapeutic strategies in SMA can be divided into those targeting SMN protein and those independent of SMN. The latter can be further divided into eight different therapeutic approaches Fig. (**3**). The fact that *SMN2* copies can produce a variable amount of SMN protein to compensate for the lack of a functioning *SMN1* in SMA provided an initial therapeutic target for attempting to augment the *SMN2* function to increase SMN protein [54]. This approach was successful by the initial proof-of-concept studies [55, 56]. Meanwhile, increasing evidence has shown that SMN deficiency produced pathology beyond MNs and involved cells both within and outside the CNS. Pathological changes have been identified in several peripheral organs, such as the cardiovascular system, gastrointestinal tract, immune system, and kidneys, both in pre-clinical animal models and in SMA patients [20, 50, 57 - 60].

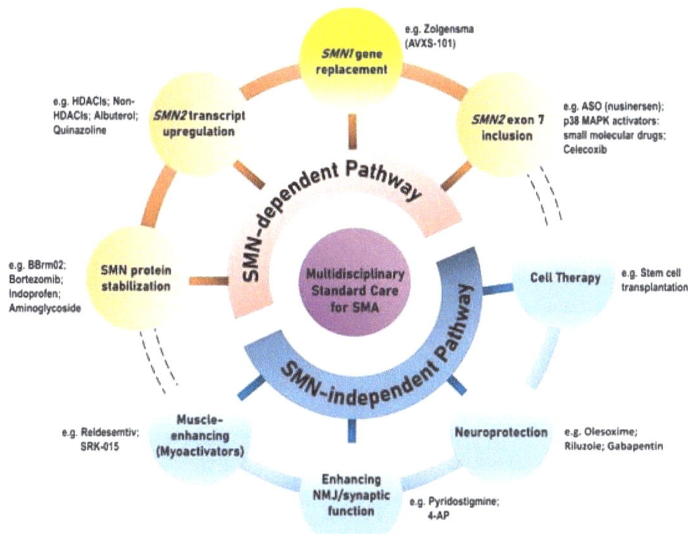

Fig. (3). Therapeutic approaches for SMA [30].

We summary the updated information of pre-clinical and clinical trials for potential therapeutic agents in Table **2**. Understanding the precise underlying mechanisms of whether the therapy relies on SMN-dependent or SMN-independent pathways remains an essential aspect of therapeutic development for SMA [61]. Among these therapeutic approaches, upregulating SMN protein production by modulating *SMN2* splicing or replacing an exogenous *SMN1* gene has proven the most successful [62, 63]. These two forms of therapeutics have been introduced into commercial use after approved by the FDA over the past two years. Parallel to these SMN-dependent approaches, several SMN-independent therapeutics such as neuroprotective agents, myostatin inhibitors, skeletal muscle troponin activator, and stem cell therapy are being developed as possible adjunctive therapies [64, 65]. Importantly, the recent breakthrough of novel therapies for SMA may also inspire similar approaches for other genetic MND. For example, spinal muscular atrophy with respiratory distress type 1 (SMARD1) caused by *IGHMBP2* gene mutation is a non-5q SMA, which accounts for the second most common MND of infancy following SMA [66].

In the following sections, we will describe the therapeutic development of several SMN-dependent compounds and the status of several SMN-independent targeting treatments aiming at both CNS and-non-CNS tissues.

The therapeutic approaches for SMA are generally categorized into SMN-dependent and SMN-independent therapies, which can be further divided into four branches of development, respectively. The yellow circle color of *SMN1* gene replacement therapy of SMN-dependent pathway indicates its difference from other three therapies in the SMN-dependent category which mainly target *SMN2*. The dash lines of outer rims connecting the SMN-dependent and SMN-independent approaches imply the potential for combinatory effect as a "cocktail therapy" for SMA.

SMN-DEPENDENT THERAPIES FOR SMA

SMA has been regarded as a unique model disease for translational research due to its well understood molecular pathogenesis and a clear therapeutic target of *SMN2* gene retained in all SMA patients. As a proof-of-concept, the initial approach was to modify *SMN2* gene expression in order to increase the FL-SMN transcripts to replace the function of the missing *SMN1* gene [1, 3, 29, 50]. As shown in Table **2**, this idea prompted investigations into the upregulation of *SMN2* transcription by activating promoter of the gene, enhancing exon 7 inclusion during splicing, modulating SMN protein translation, and preventing SMN protein degradation. Another way of replacing the *SMN1* gene function would be to introduce an exogenous *SMN1* gene *via* a viral vector directly.

Previous SMN-Targeted Clinical Trials with Equivocal Outcomes

Early studies investigating the therapeutic potential of histone deacetylase inhibitors (HDACIs) and demonstrated their ability to increase *SMN2* transcription through modification of chromatin structure *in vitro* and in SMA animal models [56, 67]. Histones are core proteins of chromatin that play a role in epigenetic regulation of gene expression *via* their acetylation status. Several potential HDACIs were initially proposed to benefit SMA, including valproic acid, phenylbutyrate, and trichostatin A, which activated the *SMN2* promotor and increased the FL-SMN production [65, 68].

Table 2. Novel therapeutic approaches in spinal muscular atrophy: Current clinical trials and preclinical strategies.

Category of Therapeutic Approach	Compound (Drug)	Therapeutic Approach (Mechanism of Action)	Clinical Phase	Sponsor	Trials for Patients' SMA type	Identifier(s)
SMN-Dependent Approach						
Replacement of *SMN1*	Zolgensma (AVXS-101)	Virus-vector *SMN1* transfer	FDA-Approved	AveXis/Novartis	1,2,3 pre-symptomatic	NCT02122952 NCT03306277 NCT03381729 NCT03421977 NCT03461289 NCT03505099 NCT04042025
Enhancing *SMN2* exon 7 inclusion	Nusinersen (Spinraza; ISIS-SMNRx; ISIS 396443)	Promotion of exon 7 inclusion by suppressing intronic splicing silencer	FDA-Approved	Biogen/Ionis	1,2,3 pre-symptomatic	NCT02052791 NCT02386553 NCT01703988 NCT01780246 NCT02292537 NCT02462759 NCT02865109 NCT02594124 NCT02193074 NCT01839656 NCT03339830 NCT01494701 NCT03709784
	Risdiplam (RG7916; RO7034067)	*SMN2* Splicing modulator	Phases 2/3, active	Roche-Genetech/PTC	1,2,3 pre-symptomatic	NCT02633709 NCT02913482 NCT02908685 NCT03032172 NCT03779334 NCT03988907
	Branaplam (LMI070)	*SMN2* Splicing modulator through U1 snRNP interaction pathway	Phase 1/2, active	Novartis	1	NCT02268552
	RG7800	*SMN2* Splicing modulator	suspended	Hoffmann-La Roche	1,2,3	NCT02240355
SMN2 transcript upregulation	Celecoxib	Cyclooxygenase 2 inhibitor to modulate *SMN2* Splicing through p38 pathway activation	Phase 2, Recruiting	Hugh McMillan	2,3	NCT02876094
	Quinazoline (RG3039)	A DcpS inhibitor to stabilize *SMN2* mRNA by modulating metabolism of RNA	suspended	Cure SMA	-	-
Stabilization of SMN protein	BBrm02	Stop codon Read-through (azithromycin)	Preclinical	BioBlast Pharma	-	-
	Bortezomib	Proteasome inhibitors	Preclinical	-	-	-

Category of Therapeutic Approach	Compound (Drug)	Therapeutic Approach (Mechanism of Action)	Clinical Phase	Sponsor	Trials for Patients' SMA type	Identifier(s)
SMN-Independent Approach						
Neuroprotection	Olesoxime (TRO19622)	Neuroprotection	Suspended	Roche-Genentech	2,3	NCT02628743
Muscle-enhancing (Myoactivators)	SRK-015	Myostatin inhibitor	Phase 2, recruiting	Scholar Rock	2,3	NCT03921528
	Reldesemtiv (CK-2127107)	Skeletal muscle troponin activation	Phase 2, completed	Cytokinetics/ Astellas	2,3,4	NCT02644668
	BIIB110	Both myostatin and activins inhibitor	Phase 1a, recruiting	Biogen	Healthy individuals	-
Enhancing function of neuromuscular junction or synaptic	Pyridostigmine	Anticholinesterase	Phase 2, completed	UMC Utrecht	2, 3, 4	NCT02227823 NCT02941328
	4-aminopyridine (4-AP) (Ampyra)	Acetylcholinesterase inhibitor	Phase 2/3, completed	Columbia University	3,4	NCT01645787
Cell Therapy using stem cells	Neural Stem Cells; Embryonic Stem Cells; Induced Pluripotent Stem Cells	Neurotrophic Support Regeneration of motor neuron	Preclinical		-	-

SMN: survival motor neuron; FDA: Food and Drug Administration

However, despite these encouraging observations *in vitro,* no beneficial effect of HDACIs was carried over to clinical trials [69]. Also, it seems that HDACIs actions are not specific to the *SMN2* gene. Its potential side effects also limited the therapeutic dose ranges [67, 70].

Besides histone acetylation, several other molecular mechanisms such as histone phosphorylation, ubiquitination, and DNA methylation, also affect *SMN2* expression [77]. Hydroxyurea, an FDA approved compound used for neoplasms and anemia, was identified in the course of drug screen using cell lines from SMA patients to increase the amount of FL-SMN transcript and protein *in vitro* [72]. However, a small pilot study of hydroxyurea at three different doses for eight weeks in 33 patients with types 2 and 3 SMA patients showed no statistically significant benefit [73]. A randomized, double-blind, placebo-controlled trial failed to show any clinical improvement over 18 months [74].

Albuterol, a β- adrenergic agonist, was able to increase FL-SMN transcript levels in severe SMA patient-derived cell lines [75]. In a pilot study of patients with types 2 and 3 SMA, treatment with albuterol led to an increase in FL-SMN transcripts and improvement of motor function with no severe side effect [76]. Another pilot study treating 23 patients with type 2 SMA with salbutamol, a form of albuterol, also demonstrated improved motor function [77]. However, there has been no data from a larger placebo-controlled trial to support the use of albuterol in clinical practice for SMA [65].

These early SMN-targeted trials, including valproic acid combined with acetyl-L-carnitine, phenylbutyrate, hydroxyurea, and somatotropin, despite their promising pre-clinical data, showed negative results following clinical trials. Their further development was discontinued except albuterol, which is still broadly prescribed off-label. However, through these negative studies, researchers have gained substantial experience in the areas of clinical trial design and development and validation of specific outcome measures [50, 78].

Nusinersen: The First Approved Splicing-Modify Therapy for SMA

In 2006, researchers discovered that an intronic splicing silencer N1 (ISS-N1) sequence in intron 7 of *SMN2* is involved in the skipping of exon 7 during mRNA splicing and produces an *SMN2* transcript lacking exon 7 (SMNΔ7) [79]. Subsequent studies found that inhibition of ISS-N1 motifs through antisense oligonucleotides (ASOs) could enhance the inclusion of exon 7 during *SMN2* transcription and rescued the severe phenotype ina s SMA animal model [80 - 83].

Among different types of ASOs, nusinersen (or Spinraza™ or ISIS-SMNRx), a 2'-O-methoxyethyl phosphorothioate-modified ASO, was found to be able to inhibit ISS-N1 most efficiently and produced functional SMN. In 2011, the phase 1 trial demonstrated the safety and efficacy of nusinersen through direct administration into the cerebrospinal fluid (CSF) space of the spinal cord in twenty-eight patients with types 2 and 3 SMA [84]. These trials were followed by phase 2 [85], and a further phase 3, multicenter, double-blind, placebo-controlled trial (ENDEAR) [63]. The ENDEAR trial demonstrated that nusinersen treatment resulted in a significantly more type 1 SMA infants achieving higher motor milestones and surviving without ventilatory support, compared with those in the control group. Excitingly, nusinersen became the first disease-modifying treatment to be approved by the FDA in December of 2016, and by the European Medicines Agency in June 2017. Subsequently, a phase 3 sham-controlled study on children with later-onset type 2 SMA also showed significant improvement in their motor functions [86].

To date, more than 8,000 patients with SMA have undergone therapy with nusinersen worldwide [29]. However, in addition to a $750,000 high price tag for the first year of treatment, questions about its long-term efficacy and other limitations remained. First, there is a limited therapeutic window when treatments to increase SMN levels are most effective [87]. In the ENDEAR, as mentioned above trial, the motor function was unfortunately not wholly restored in all treated type 1 SMA infants. The most significant improvements were found in those who started treatment early within 13 weeks of symptom onset [63]. This finding prompted the attempt to correlate the timing of treatment and its efficacy. This is being investigated in an ongoing phase 2 study of 25 presymptomatic, genetically-confirmed SMA infants (NURTURE Study; NCT02386553). The preliminary results from interim analysis at a median age of 2.9 years showed a hundred percent survival with unsupported sitting, and 88% of independent walking [88]. These findings highlight the importance of a therapeutic window for an SMN-augmented treatment. Unfortunately, SMA newborn screening program has not yet extensively performed worldwide or even nationwide [89, 90]. On the other hand, patients with later-onset type 2 SMA showed significant motor improvement after treatment [86]. It is not clear if any therapeutic effect can be seen when this *SMN2*-targeted ASO therapy is given at the severe stage of the disease when there are very few MNs left within the spinal cord [91]. The temporal requirements for SMN protein in other non-neuronal tissues are even less understood [92].

Second limitation is the route of administration. Because nusinersen cannot penetrate the blood-brain barrier (BBB) to reach the MNs, there is no practical alternative to periodic intrathecal administration. The risks of performing lumbar puncture in SMA patients include exacerbating respiratory distress during the procedure and headache associated with CSF leakage after the procedure. Moreover, repetitive intrathecal injections can present challenges in some chronic SMA patients with significant scoliosis or those who have had spinal fusions [92]. Use of computed-tomography guidance, videofluorangiography, ultrasound-guided, and novel techniques like subcutaneous intrathecal catheters are options to consider in such cases, but potential complications of these procedures have not been well studied [93, 94].

The third consideration is that SMN protein may be needed in peripheral tissues in addition to the spinal cord MNs. Emerging evidence suggested that SMN plays a vital role in peripheral tissues [95, 96]. Hua *et al.* reported a marked improvement in motor function and survival after systemic delivery of ASO 1 in the Taiwanese SMA mice. They found increased SMN protein in several peripheral tissues, especially in the liver [97]. They further demonstrated that peripheral SMN restoration compensates for its deficiency in the CNS and preserves MNs [98]. These findings suggest an essential role of peripheral tissues in SMA pathogenesis. The study of the impact of low SMN levels on other organ systems such as cardiovascular, gastrointestinal, or immune systems may reveal an unsuspected vulnerability in these organs [92]. To date, the safety of the systemic ASO delivery in humans is still under evaluation.

Gene Therapy for SMA: *SMN1* Gene Replacement

Another way to augment SMN production in the MNs can be achieved by directly transferring the *SMN1* gene into the cell. Theoretically, gene transfer therapy requires a vector, a transgene, and a promoter. Both lentivirus and adeno-associated viral (AAV) vectors have been used to deliver the *SMN1* gene to the SMN-defected MNs. However, lack of specific affinity to neuronal cell and inability to pass BBB render the lentivirus less suitable for use as an *SMN1* gene delivering vector [99, 100]. The immunogenic reaction by the recipient host was another concern. The self-complementary adeno-associated virus 9 (scAAV9) obtained the ability to cross the BBB and infected approximately 60% of MNs when injected intravenously into neonatal mice [101 - 103]. The additional advantages of lower immunogenicity and large packaging capacity render scAAV9 to be an ideal vector [104, 105]. The packed genome is designed with a hybrid cytomegalovirus enhancer-chicken beta-actin promoter- to drive high, sustained human *SMN1* expression. This novelty was achieved by increasing the initiation of transgene translation, avoiding the rate-limiting step of cell-mediated second-strand synthesis typically required by recombinant AAV, and promoting rapid and efficient transduction [106]. The efficacy of SMN1 replacement therapy was subsequently proved by an *in vivo* study using an SMNΔ7 murine model. The study showed that postnatal intravenous gene therapy using the *SMN1* packaged viral vector rescued their motor function and extended survival from 2 weeks to beyond 250 days [101].

Excitingly, a phase 1/2a trial of Zolgensma (also known as AVXS-101 and onasemnogene abeparvovec) studying 15 patients with type 1 SMA, receiving either a low dose (6.7×10^{13} vg/Kg) or high dose (2×10^{14} vg/Kg) of transferred *SMN1* gene, showed that all patients were alive at least 20 months of age [62]. Similar to patients who received nusinersen therapy, the long-term follow-up study also showed that infants with early gene therapy achieved motor milestones much faster than those who received the therapy late [107]. Zolgensma was approved by the FDA on May 24, 2019, for treating SMA patients younger than 2-year-old.

The promising results of this phase 1/2a trial of Zolgensma are currently further evaluated in open-label, single-arm phase 3 trials on type 1 SMA infants (<6 months old) with 1 or 2 *SMN2* copies (STR1VE; NCT03306277 in the US and NCT03461289 in EU). The preliminary data continue to demonstrate promising results [108, 109]. Another phase 3 global trial (SPR1NT; NCT03505099) evaluating drug efficacy in presymptomatic infants with SMA (≤ 6 weeks old) is currently ongoing and still enrolling patients [102]. However, the FDA has recently placed a partial hold on the intrathecal administration of Zolgensma

(STRONG, NCT03381729) in older SMA patients ($\geq$ 2 years and < 5 years) based on safety concerns from a small pre-clinical animal study [110].

Because of different study designs, it is hard to compare the efficacies between these FDA-approved ASO-based and gene-based SMA therapies. However, the mean age of the patients was slightly lower in the Zolgensma trial than in the nusinersen trial (3.4 months *vs.* 5.4 months). There are several advantages of scAAV9-based gene therapy potentially superior to ASO SMN-augmentation therapy [111]. First, scAAV9 gene therapy has a sustainable effect and may only require a single dose of intravenous infusion, whereas nusinersen may require lifelong intrathecal treatment. Second, given that SMN protein is ubiquitously expressed, systemic delivery of the AAV-vector packaged *SMN1* gene through the intravenous route has the advantage of increasing SMN expression in other organ systems in the body [29].

Nevertheless, there are still several concerns to be addressed, as recent studies showed AAV9-*SMN* gene therapy administered through the intravenous route in large animals have suboptimal outcomes [112, 113]. One of the notable concerns of AAV9-based gene therapy is the ubiquitous expression of SMN, leading to the nonspecific sequestration of essential RNAs and proteins through RNA-protein and protein-protein interactions. Furthermore, poor body-wide delivery of viral particles was observed. The potential immune response to the viral vector by the treated hosts remains a concern for gene replacement therapy [114].

Other Small-Molecule SMN Splicing Modifiers

Several small molecules currently under investigation in pre-clinical studies or clinical trials provided an encouraging landscape for the development of alternative or complementary SMA therapy. The oral bioavailability with a promising potential to reach various tissues systemically makes these novel small-molecule drugs quite attractive as candidates for SMA treatment. Highly specific interactions between small molecules and the unique RNA structures of *SMN2* pre-mRNA have been considered as the advantage in the correction of exon 7 splicings of *SMN2* transcripts. Considering the complex network and the unique molecular structures associated with *SMN2* pre-mRNA, the potential to identify additional RNA-structure-interacting, small molecules for specific splicing correction remains very high.

Risdiplam (RG7916)

RG7800 is a small molecule that initially brought hope for these groups of drugs to SMA treatment [115]. In a phase 1 trial (MOONFISH; NCT02240355), no serious adverse events were reported following oral administration of RG7800 in patients with types 2 and 3 SMA. However, further study was suspended due to offtarget retinal findings in longterm, nonclinical safety studies in monkeys [116]. Subsequently, Risdiplam (RG7916), an RG7800-like but structure modified compound, also shows a comparative ability to enhance the inclusion of *SMN2* exon 7 during mRNA splicing. Risdiplam demonstrated a higher *in vitro* and *in vivo* efficacy in cellular and SMA mouse models with a more extensive safety window (including the offtarget retinal findings) and an improved human pharmacokinetic (PK) profile compared with RG7800 [117]. Risdiplam increases FL-*SMN2* transcripts in the CNS and peripheral tissues by avoiding interaction with human multidrug resistance protein 1 (MDR1), a transporter protein that restricts brain exposure. The potential of being able to distribute to both CNS and peripheral tissues makes Risdiplam a compelling therapeutic candidate to treat SMA as a whole-body disease [118]. Both trials recruiting patients with type 1 SMA aged 1-7 months (FIREFISH), and patients with types 2 and 3 aged 2-25 years (SUNFISH), demonstrated positive results. Those tested patients showed not only a significant increment of SMN protein in blood but also improvement in motor functions with event-free survival [119 - 121]. Another trial (JEWELFISH; NCT03032172) is currently ongoing in SMA types 2 and 3 patients who had been treated with other agents previously (such as RG7800 or nusinersen). The results of this study are pending.

Branaplam (LMI070)

Branaplam (LMI070 or NVS-SM1) works by stabilizing *SMN2* and U1 snRNP interaction to facilitate exon 7 inclusion during mRNA splicing [115]. In an SMA mouse pre-clinical study, Branaplam was found to increase SMN level and to improve body weight and survival [122]. An ongoing phase 1/2, open-label, first-in-human clinical trial of Branaplam is evaluating the safety, tolerability, pharmacokinetics, pharmacodynamics, and efficacy in patients with type 1 SMA younger than eight months. The preliminary analysis of eight patients showed significant improvement in motor function with an excellent safety profile after 86 days of treatment. After 127 days of treatment, five patients still showed persistent improvement [123].

Celecoxib

Treatment with celecoxib, a cyclooxygenase 2 inhibitor, increased SMN RNA and protein levels *in vitro*. In models of severe SMA mice, it activated the p38 pathway and might have a neuroprotective effect by inhibition of glutamate release [124]. Several factors make the celecoxib appealing as a treatment for human SMA patients. These include (1) low-dosing required for potential therapeutic effect, (2) favorable side effect profile, and (3) the fact that celecoxib crosses the BBB. A phase 2 open-label trial in children and adults with SMA types 2 and 3 is actively recruiting patients to investigate the effect of different dosages of celecoxib on SMN protein levels in peripheral leukocytes [65]. It may be with the hope that celecoxib may serve as adjunctive therapy for SMA, particularly given the low safe doses are required for SMN induction.

Quinazoline (Repligen RG3039)

Blocking of decapping scavenger enzyme (DcpS) shows to increase in the FL-*SMN2* transcript through upregulating *SMN2* promoter activity [125]. Quinazoline (Repligen or RG3039), a DcpS inhibitor, demonstrated to increase in SMN protein and survival in SMA mice [126]. However, a phase 1b trial showed that even though RG3039 successfully blocked DcpS in patients' blood, the SMN protein level did not change significantly [127]. Therefore, the pharmaceutic company concluded that RG3039 would be ineffective in SMA patients, and the further trial was halted [128].

Full-Length SMN Protein Stabilizer

Aminoglycoside antibiotics (from a class of FDA-approved drugs including tobramycin, geneticin, and amikacin) can mask premature stop codon mutations and promote read-through of exon 8, and thereby stabilize or increase the SMN level in SMA patients' fibroblasts [129, 130]. Various aminoglycosides, including tobramycin and amikacin, have been used successfully in SMA patient fibroblasts to increase SMN protein levels. However, no *in vivo* efficacy has been shown, and the toxicity has only been tested in animal models of SMA [70].

BBrm2 is a repurposed FDA-approved azithromycin acting on stop codon read-through. It has been found to increase SMN protein in human SMA cell lines, and improved motor function and survival when intrathecally delivered to an SMA mouse [70]. The positive results have also been shown in another SMA mouse model [131].

Bortezomib is a ubiquitin-proteasome inhibitor known to prevent SMN protein degradation. It was shown to increases SMN protein in cultured cells and peripheral tissues of SMA model mice. Bortezomib-treated animals had improved motor function with reduced spinal cord and muscle pathology and improved neuromuscular junction morphology but no change in survival [132].

SMN-INDEPENDENT THERAPIES FOR SMA

As the first successful SMN-targeted therapeutics are emerging into the clinical arena, other approaches beyond SMN augmentation are also under active investigation. It is agreed that the SMN-targeted treatments should be initiated as early as possible to maximize the therapeutic effects. However, this may not be possible for those with chronic forms (types 3 and 4) of SMA, who are often diagnosed after the substantial loss of MNs [133]. Instead of trying to catch the therapeutic windows, it may be more crucial to target the SMN-independent pathways that are often disrupted downstream of SMN. Besides, emerging evidence has shown that SMA is a systemic disorder that goes beyond MNs. Therefore, further development and implementation of SMN-independent therapies are incredibly relevant, considering that SMN-dependent approaches only lessen the disease severity but do not cure the disease [29, 134].

Since treatments for SMA are likely to last for the entire life span, and both SMN-dependent and SMN-independent therapies have been shown beneficial, a combination of both forms of therapies are likely to be used in these patients. For these reasons, considerable effort has gone into developing therapies that do not depend on raising SMN levels. In the following sections, we will discuss how the current non-SMN-targeted compounds are being developed through clinical trials and discuss the potential applications of these SMN-independent approaches in protecting non-CNS tissues.

Neuroprotective Agents

Olesoxime (TRO19622) is a member of the trophos cholesterol-oxime compound family of mitochondrial pore modulators with neuroprotective properties. Pre-clinical studies suggest that it improves the function and survival of neurons [135]. A phase 2 placebo-controlled trial in patients with types 2 and 3 SMA showed stabilized motor function at 24 months of treatment [136]. However, subsequent follow-up study at 18 months did not demonstrate a significant clinical benefit (OLEOS, NCT02628743), and the pharmaceutical company announced to end the development of olesoxime for SMA in June 2018 [29].

Other neuroprotective agents such as riluzole and gabapentin have been investigated for their effects in treating SMA [137, 138]. A phase 2/3 multicenter, randomized, double-blind study to assess the efficacy and safety of riluzole in young adults with types 2 and 3 SMA has been completed. Unfortunately, the results were not encouraging, and no treatment efficacy was demonstrated [1, 65].

Myostatin Inhibitors

Since muscle weakness is always associated with SMA, some of the new SMN-independent therapies have focused on strengthening the muscle. Myostatin is a growth factor produced primarily in skeletal muscle cells to inhibit muscle growth. Theoretically, blocking the myostatin signaling pathway can increase muscle mass and improve muscle strength and motor function [139]. Follistatin is an endogenous antagonist of myostatin, and over-expression of recombinant follistatin in SMA mouse muscle leads to increased skeletal muscle mass as well as survival [140].

On the other hand, inhibition of activin receptor type IIB (ActRIIB) ligands can promote muscle growth, which suggests a potential therapy for neuromuscular disorders, including SMA. Systemic delivery of AAV-mediated soluble inhibitor of ActRIIB showed improvements both in muscle mass and muscle function of the SMA mouse model [141]. BIIB 110 (ALG 801) is a recombinant inhibitor of ActRIIB, which is undergoing a phase 1a trial [142].

Another myostatin inhibitor, SRK-015 (Scholar Rock), is a human monoclonal antibody found to increase muscle mass in SMA mice [143]. A phase 2 trial in type 2 and type 3 SMA patients through monthly intravenous administration is underway (TOPAZ; NCT03921528), and the preliminary data demonstrated a robust and dose-dependent target engagement on myostatin precursor [144].

Skeletal Muscle Troponin Activator: Reldesemtiv

Reldesemtiv (CK-2127107) is a fast skeletal muscle troponin activator, which has shown to improve muscle function and physical performance in SMA [70]. Reldesemtiv demonstrated to increase in skeletal muscle force in response to nerve stimulation, associated with a calcium-sensitizing effect [145]. The initial human trial showed promising results with prolonged stamina and modest improvement in pulmonary function [146]. This prompted an ongoing double-blind phase 2 clinical trial to examine the efficacy of orally given twice a day in non-type 1 SMA patients (>12 years old) who are either ambulatory or non-ambulatory (NCT02644668) [147].

Agents Targeting Neuromuscular Junction, Synapse, or Neurotransmitter

Pyridostigmine

Pyridostigmine (Mestinon) is approved in the U.S. and Europe as a first-line treatment for myasthenia gravis. Pyridostigmine prevents the enzyme acetylcholinesterase from breaking down acetylcholine — a chemical messenger (neurotransmitter) released by MNs to activate muscle contractions. Treatment of pyridostigmine raises the concentration and prolongs the action of acetylcholine in the neuromuscular junctions, thereby, enhances the transmission of nerve impulses to muscles. Researchers believe that the medicine's ability to activate and strengthen muscles might benefit SMA patients [148]. The randomized, placebo-controlled, double-blind trial, named SPACE, is currently investigating the effects of pyridostigmine on muscle strength and fatigue in 39 patients with types 2-4 SMA [149].

4-aminopyridine

4-aminopyridine (4-AP or Ampyra) is an FDA-approved drug developed by Acorda Therapeutics for the treatment of multiple sclerosis. 4-AP is a broad-spectrum inhibitor of potassium channels, which improves the phenotypes of the SMA Drosophila, possibly through the pathway of influencing motor circuitry [150]. Although not yet tested in the SMA mouse model, a phase 2/3 trial assessing the efficacy in walking ability and motor endurance in 18- to 50- year-olds SMA type 3 patients had been completed in 2017, but the results have not yet been published [151].

Stem Cells Therapy

The rationale of cell therapy in SMA is mainly related to their ability to replace the degenerating MNs. Interest in the use of stem cells also continued, both as a potential treatment of SMA and for use in constructing model systems for therapeutics development. Pluripotent stem cells with the capacity to differentiate into MNs lacking *SMN1* expression were induced from a patient with type 1 SMA and his mother. This technique could serve as an important model system for testing new compounds and eventually for stem cell transplant to the treatment of SMA [152].

Two currently available stem cell transplantation studies in SMA mice showed that primary motor neuron stem cells injected into the spinal canal engrafted to the spinal cord, improved motor function and extended survival by 39% [153, 154]. However, these results likely only reflected benefits from trophic support without evidence of functional cell replacement. While the progress of pre-clinical stem cell research for SMA seems promising, validation of their therapeutic efficacy and knowledge on the mechanism of action is still lacking.

COMBINATION THERAPY FOR SMA

The concept that a combination of different therapeutic strategies could maximize the benefits for SMA treatment is intriguing. Although combined therapies with expensive drugs may, at some point, be prohibitive and limited data, support the efficacy of such combination on human, physicians, and scientists are encouraged to explore all therapeutic possibilities [155]. On a positive note, encouraging evidence has shown that the combined SMN-dependent approach of ASO-inducing *SMN2* exon inclusion and SMN-independent approach of myostatin inhibition in an SMA animal model have shown a favorable result [156].

Combined treatment with Zolgensma and Nusinersen has been recently investigated in a small group of patients, but the long-term benefit is still unclear [157]. Zolgensma and nusinersen have different mechanisms of action, and the drug-to-drug interaction is expected to be minimal. Nusinersen ASO affects the transcription of *SMN2* mRNA, targeting an intron sequence to enhance exon 7 inclusion. The AAV9-*SMN1* transgene does not contain any introns, so its translation should not be affected by the presence of Nusinersen [134]. Due to thrombocytopenia has been reported as an adverse event in association with nusinersen, caution is required when Zolgensma treatment is considered. Longer-term follow-up data, especially in the treatment of presymptomatic patients, should be accumulated to assess efficacy and risks of combination therapy.

CONCLUSIONS

Although there are now two approved therapies for SMA targeting the SMN-dependent pathway, it is clear that neither treatment enables a complete cure. Ongoing research is continuing to identify more potential treatments through the development of novel compounds. Each of the treatments mentioned above can potentially be a promising treatment for SMA. However, discovering novel therapeutics relies on a better understanding of SMA pathogenetic mechanisms, the natural history, and the ongoing impact of multidisciplinary care.

With the availability of the disease-modifying therapies, the SMA phenotypes are expected to be significantly altered. We are anticipating to encounter a new group of disease modified patients with extended life expectancy, even within the most severe phenotype. Some of them will continue to exhibit significant disability and continue to require comprehensive multidisciplinary care. Some of the type 1 SMA patients may live to adulthood, and new symptoms in other organ systems that were never observed before may evolve and become evident. The medical community will need to continue to assess the different needs of this new group of SMA patients and provide timely assessment and treatment. With the increasing number of therapies available for SMA, decisions about the selection of different treatment options and how to make them available to the patients should be topics of ongoing discussion among all stakeholders (industry, the health-care system, patients, and caregivers). Patient support groups such as SMA Foundation, CureSMA, and Fight SMA, as well as the SMA families and their caregivers, have played vital roles in the past, and their support will continue to be needed for the ongoing research efforts in order to advance the SMA therapy.

CONSENT FOR PUBLICATION

Not Applicable.

CONFLICT OF INTEREST

The author confirms that the content of this chapter has no conflict of interest.

ACKNOWLEDGEMENTS

None declared.

REFERENCES

[1]   Darras BT. Spinal muscular atrophies. Pediatr Clin North Am 2015; 62(3): 743-66.
        [http://dx.doi.org/10.1016/j.pcl.2015.03.010] [PMID: 26022173]

[2]   Kolb SJ, Kissel JT. Spinal muscular atrophy: a timely review. Arch Neurol 2011; 68(8): 979-84.
        [http://dx.doi.org/10.1001/archneurol.2011.74] [PMID: 21482919]

[3]   Lunn MR, Wang CH. Spinal muscular atrophy. Lancet 2008; 371(9630): 2120-33.
        [http://dx.doi.org/10.1016/S0140-6736(08)60921-6] [PMID: 18572081]

[4]   Dubowitz V. Ramblings in the history of spinal muscular atrophy. Neuromuscul Disord 2009; 19(1):
        69-73.
        [http://dx.doi.org/10.1016/j.nmd.2008.10.004] [PMID: 18951794]

[5]   Lefebvre S, Bürglen L, Reboullet S, *et al.* Identification and characterization of a spinal muscular
        atrophy-determining gene. Cell 1995; 80(1): 155-65.
        [http://dx.doi.org/10.1016/0092-8674(95)90460-3] [PMID: 7813012]

[6]   Coovert DD, Le TT, McAndrew PE, *et al.* The survival motor neuron protein in spinal muscular
        atrophy. Hum Mol Genet 1997; 6(8): 1205-14.
        [http://dx.doi.org/10.1093/hmg/6.8.1205] [PMID: 9259265]

[7]   Singh RN, Howell MD, Ottesen EW, Singh NN. Diverse role of survival motor neuron protein.
        Biochim Biophys Acta Gene Regul Mech 2017; 1860(3): 299-315.
        [http://dx.doi.org/10.1016/j.bbagrm.2016.12.008] [PMID: 28095296]

[8]   Dostie J, Mourelatos Z, Yang M, Sharma A, Dreyfuss G. Numerous microRNPs in neuronal cells
        containing novel microRNAs. RNA 2003; 9(2): 180-6.
        [http://dx.doi.org/10.1261/rna.2141503] [PMID: 12554860]

[9]   Burghes AH, Beattie CE. Spinal muscular atrophy: why do low levels of survival motor neuron
        protein make motor neurons sick? Nat Rev Neurosci 2009; 10(8): 597-609.
        [http://dx.doi.org/10.1038/nrn2670] [PMID: 19584893]

[10]   Chaytow H, Huang YT, Gillingwater TH, Faller KME. The role of survival motor neuron protein
        (SMN) in protein homeostasis. Cell Mol Life Sci 2018; 75(21): 3877-94.
        [http://dx.doi.org/10.1007/s00018-018-2849-1] [PMID: 29872871]

[11]   Meister G, Fischer U. Assisted RNP assembly: SMN and PRMT5 complexes cooperate in the
        formation of spliceosomal UsnRNPs. EMBO J 2002; 21(21): 5853-63.
        [http://dx.doi.org/10.1093/emboj/cdf585] [PMID: 12411503]

[12]   Pellizzoni L, Baccon J, Rappsilber J, Mann M, Dreyfuss G. Purification of native survival of motor
        neurons complexes and identification of Gemin6 as a novel component. J Biol Chem 2002; 277(9):
        7540-5.
        [http://dx.doi.org/10.1074/jbc.M110141200] [PMID: 11748230]

[13]   Gabanella F, Butchbach ME, Saieva L, Carissimi C, Burghes AH, Pellizzoni L. Ribonucleoprotein
        assembly defects correlate with spinal muscular atrophy severity and preferentially affect a subset of
        spliceosomal snRNPs. PLoS One 2007; 2(9): e921.
        [http://dx.doi.org/10.1371/journal.pone.0000921] [PMID: 17895963]

[14] Workman E, Saieva L, Carrel TL, *et al.* A SMN missense mutation complements SMN2 restoring snRNPs and rescuing SMA mice. Hum Mol Genet 2009; 18(12): 2215-29.
[http://dx.doi.org/10.1093/hmg/ddp157] [PMID: 19329542]

[15] Winkler C, Eggert C, Gradl D, *et al.* Reduced U snRNP assembly causes motor axon degeneration in an animal model for spinal muscular atrophy. Genes Dev 2005; 19(19): 2320-30.
[http://dx.doi.org/10.1101/gad.342005] [PMID: 16204184]

[16] Jodelka FM, Ebert AD, Duelli DM, Hastings ML. A feedback loop regulates splicing of the spinal muscular atrophy-modifying gene, SMN2. Hum Mol Genet 2010; 19(24): 4906-17.
[http://dx.doi.org/10.1093/hmg/ddq425] [PMID: 20884664]

[17] Murray LM, Beauvais A, Gibeault S, Courtney NL, Kothary R. Transcriptional profiling of differentially vulnerable motor neurons at pre-symptomatic stage in the Smn (2b/-) mouse model of spinal muscular atrophy. Acta Neuropathol Commun 2015; 3: 55.
[http://dx.doi.org/10.1186/s40478-015-0231-1] [PMID: 26374403]

[18] Fallini C, Bassell GJ, Rossoll W. Spinal muscular atrophy: the role of SMN in axonal mRNA regulation. Brain Res 2012; 1462: 81-92.
[http://dx.doi.org/10.1016/j.brainres.2012.01.044] [PMID: 22330725]

[19] Donlin-Asp PG, Bassell GJ, Rossoll W. A role for the survival of motor neuron protein in mRNP assembly and transport. Curr Opin Neurobiol 2016; 39: 53-61.
[http://dx.doi.org/10.1016/j.conb.2016.04.004] [PMID: 27131421]

[20] Hamilton G, Gillingwater TH. Spinal muscular atrophy: going beyond the motor neuron. Trends Mol Med 2013; 19(1): 40-50.
[http://dx.doi.org/10.1016/j.molmed.2012.11.002] [PMID: 23228902]

[21] Tu WY, Simpson JE, Highley JR, Heath PR. Spinal muscular atrophy: Factors that modulate motor neurone vulnerability. Neurobiol Dis 2017; 102: 11-20.
[http://dx.doi.org/10.1016/j.nbd.2017.01.011] [PMID: 28161391]

[22] Rindt H, Feng Z, Mazzasette C, *et al.* Astrocytes influence the severity of spinal muscular atrophy. Hum Mol Genet 2015; 24(14): 4094-102.
[http://dx.doi.org/10.1093/hmg/ddv148] [PMID: 25911676]

[23] Abati E, Citterio G, Bresolin N, Comi GP, Corti S. Glial cells involvement in spinal muscular atrophy: Could SMA be a neuroinflammatory disease? Neurobiol Dis 2020; 140104870
[http://dx.doi.org/10.1016/j.nbd.2020.104870] [PMID: 32294521]

[24] Burghes AH. When is a deletion not a deletion? When it is converted. Am J Hum Genet 1997; 61(1): 9-15.
[http://dx.doi.org/10.1086/513913] [PMID: 9245977]

[25] Swoboda KJ. SMN-targeted therapeutics for spinal muscular atrophy: are we SMArt enough yet? J Clin Invest 2014; 124(2): 487-90.
[http://dx.doi.org/10.1172/JCI74142] [PMID: 24463455]

[26] Chang JG, Jong YJ, Lin SP, *et al.* Molecular analysis of survival motor neuron (SMN) and neuronal apoptosis inhibitory protein (NAIP) genes of spinal muscular atrophy patients and their parents. Hum Genet 1997; 100(5-6): 577-81.
[http://dx.doi.org/10.1007/s004390050555] [PMID: 9341874]

[27] Prior TW, Krainer AR, Hua Y, *et al.* A positive modifier of spinal muscular atrophy in the SMN2 gene. Am J Hum Genet 2009; 85(3): 408-13.
[http://dx.doi.org/10.1016/j.ajhg.2009.08.002] [PMID: 19716110]

[28] Crawford TO, Paushkin SV, Kobayashi DT, *et al.* Evaluation of SMN protein, transcript, and copy number in the biomarkers for spinal muscular atrophy (BforSMA) clinical study. PLoS One 2012; 7(4): e33572.
[http://dx.doi.org/10.1371/journal.pone.0033572] [PMID: 22558076]

[29]   Wirth B, Karakaya M, Kye MJ, Mendoza-Ferreira N. Twenty-Five Years of Spinal Muscular Atrophy Research: From Phenotype to Genotype to Therapy, and What Comes Next. Annu Rev Genomics Hum Genet 2020; 21: 4.1-4.31.

[30]   Chen TH. New and Developing Therapies in Spinal Muscular Atrophy: From Genotype to Phenotype to Treatment and Where Do We Stand? Int J Mol Sci 2020; 21(9): 21.
[http://dx.doi.org/10.3390/ijms21093297] [PMID: 32392694]

[31]   Oskoui M, Levy G, Garland CJ, *et al.* The changing natural history of spinal muscular atrophy type 1. Neurology 2007; 69(20): 1931-6.
[http://dx.doi.org/10.1212/01.wnl.0000290830.40544.b9] [PMID: 17998484]

[32]   Piepers S, van der Pol WL, Brugman F, Wokke JH, van den Berg LH. Natural history of SMA IIIb: muscle strength decreases in a predictable sequence and magnitude. Neurology 2009; 72(23): 2057-8.
[http://dx.doi.org/10.1212/01.wnl.0000349698.94744.1e] [PMID: 19506238]

[33]   Farrar MA, Vucic S, Johnston HM, du Sart D, Kiernan MC. Pathophysiological insights derived by natural history and motor function of spinal muscular atrophy. J Pediatr 2013; 162(1): 155-9.
[http://dx.doi.org/10.1016/j.jpeds.2012.05.067] [PMID: 22809660]

[34]   Markowitz JA, Singh P, Darras BT. Spinal muscular atrophy: a clinical and research update. Pediatr Neurol 2012; 46(1): 1-12.
[http://dx.doi.org/10.1016/j.pediatrneurol.2011.09.001] [PMID: 22196485]

[35]   Mercuri E, Bertini E, Iannaccone ST. Childhood spinal muscular atrophy: controversies and challenges. Lancet Neurol 2012; 11(5): 443-52.
[http://dx.doi.org/10.1016/S1474-4422(12)70061-3] [PMID: 22516079]

[36]   Nadeau A, D'Anjou G, Debray G, Robitaille Y, Simard LR, Vanasse M. A newborn with spinal muscular atrophy type 0 presenting with a clinicopathological picture suggestive of myotubular myopathy. J Child Neurol 2007; 22(11): 1301-4.
[http://dx.doi.org/10.1177/0883073807307105] [PMID: 18006961]

[37]   Dubowitz V. Very severe spinal muscular atrophy (SMA type 0): an expanding clinical phenotype. Eur J Paediatr Neurol 1999; 3(2): 49-51.
[http://dx.doi.org/10.1016/S1090-3798(99)80012-9] [PMID: 10700538]

[38]   Sansone VA, Racca F, Ottonello G, *et al.* 1st Italian SMA Family Association Consensus Meeting: Management and recommendations for respiratory involvement in spinal muscular atrophy (SMA) types I-III, Rome, Italy, 30-31 January 2015. Neuromuscul Disord 2015; 25(12): 979-89.
[http://dx.doi.org/10.1016/j.nmd.2015.09.009] [PMID: 26453142]

[39]   Wijngaarde CA, Blank AC, Stam M, Wadman RI, van den Berg LH, van der Pol WL. Cardiac pathology in spinal muscular atrophy: a systematic review. Orphanet J Rare Dis 2017; 12(1): 67.
[http://dx.doi.org/10.1186/s13023-017-0613-5] [PMID: 28399889]

[40]   Bertini E, Mercuri E. Motor neuron disease: A prospective natural history study of type 1 spinal muscular atrophy. Nat Rev Neurol 2018; 14(4): 197-8.
[http://dx.doi.org/10.1038/nrneurol.2017.189] [PMID: 29348544]

[41]   Kolb SJ, Coffey CS, Yankey JW, *et al.* Natural history of infantile-onset spinal muscular atrophy. Ann Neurol 2017; 82(6): 883-91.
[http://dx.doi.org/10.1002/ana.25101] [PMID: 29149772]

[42]   Kaufmann P, McDermott MP, Darras BT, *et al.* Observational study of spinal muscular atrophy type 2 and 3: functional outcomes over 1 year. Arch Neurol 2011; 68(6): 779-86.
[http://dx.doi.org/10.1001/archneurol.2010.373] [PMID: 21320981]

[43]   Kaufmann P, McDermott MP, Darras BT, *et al.* Prospective cohort study of spinal muscular atrophy types 2 and 3. Neurology 2012; 79(18): 1889-97.
[http://dx.doi.org/10.1212/WNL.0b013e318271f7e4] [PMID: 23077013]

[44]   Piepers S, van den Berg LH, Brugman F, *et al.* A natural history study of late onset spinal muscular atrophy types 3b and 4. J Neurol 2008; 255(9): 1400-4.
[http://dx.doi.org/10.1007/s00415-008-0929-0] [PMID: 18575920]

[45]   Finkel RS, McDermott MP, Kaufmann P, *et al.* Observational study of spinal muscular atrophy type I and implications for clinical trials. Neurology 2014; 83(9): 810-7.
[http://dx.doi.org/10.1212/WNL.0000000000000741] [PMID: 25080519]

[46]   Mercuri E, Lucibello S, Perulli M, *et al.* Longitudinal natural history of type I spinal muscular atrophy: a critical review. Orphanet J Rare Dis 2020; 15(1): 84.
[http://dx.doi.org/10.1186/s13023-020-01356-1] [PMID: 32248834]

[47]   Rudnik-Schöneborn S, Berg C, Zerres K, *et al.* Genotype-phenotype studies in infantile spinal muscular atrophy (SMA) type I in Germany: implications for clinical trials and genetic counselling. Clin Genet 2009; 76(2): 168-78.
[http://dx.doi.org/10.1111/j.1399-0004.2009.01200.x] [PMID: 19780763]

[48]   Tizzano EF, Finkel RS. Spinal muscular atrophy: A changing phenotype beyond the clinical trials. Neuromuscul Disord 2017; 27(10): 883-9.
[http://dx.doi.org/10.1016/j.nmd.2017.05.011] [PMID: 28757001]

[49]   Sansone VA, Pirola A, Albamonte E, *et al.* Respiratory Needs in Patients with Type 1 Spinal Muscular Atrophy Treated with Nusinersen. J Pediatr 2020; 219: 8-223.e4

[50]   Farrar MA, Park SB, Vucic S, *et al.* Emerging therapies and challenges in spinal muscular atrophy. Ann Neurol 2017; 81(3): 355-68.
[http://dx.doi.org/10.1002/ana.24864] [PMID: 28026041]

[51]   Wang CH, Finkel RS, Bertini ES, *et al.* Consensus statement for standard of care in spinal muscular atrophy. J Child Neurol 2007; 22(8): 1027-49.
[http://dx.doi.org/10.1177/0883073807305788] [PMID: 17761659]

[52]   Mercuri E, Finkel RS, Muntoni F, *et al.* Diagnosis and management of spinal muscular atrophy: Part 1: Recommendations for diagnosis, rehabilitation, orthopedic and nutritional care. Neuromuscul Disord 2018; 28(2): 103-15.
[http://dx.doi.org/10.1016/j.nmd.2017.11.005] [PMID: 29290580]

[53]   Finkel RS, Mercuri E, Meyer OH, *et al.* Diagnosis and management of spinal muscular atrophy: Part 2: Pulmonary and acute care; medications, supplements and immunizations; other organ systems; and ethics. Neuromuscul Disord 2018; 28(3): 197-207.
[http://dx.doi.org/10.1016/j.nmd.2017.11.004] [PMID: 29305137]

[54]   Feldkötter M, Schwarzer V, Wirth R, Wienker TF, Wirth B. Quantitative analyses of SMN1 and SMN2 based on real-time lightCycler PCR: fast and highly reliable carrier testing and prediction of severity of spinal muscular atrophy. Am J Hum Genet 2002; 70(2): 358-68.
[http://dx.doi.org/10.1086/338627] [PMID: 11791208]

[55]   Burnett BG, Crawford TO, Sumner CJ. Emerging treatment options for spinal muscular atrophy. Curr Treat Options Neurol 2009; 11(2): 90-101.
[http://dx.doi.org/10.1007/s11940-009-0012-x] [PMID: 19210911]

[56]   Chang JG, Hsieh-Li HM, Jong YJ, Wang NM, Tsai CH, Li H. Treatment of spinal muscular atrophy by sodium butyrate. Proc Natl Acad Sci USA 2001; 98(17): 9808-13.
[http://dx.doi.org/10.1073/pnas.171105098] [PMID: 11504946]

[57]   Schreml J, Riessland M, Paterno M, *et al.* Severe SMA mice show organ impairment that cannot be rescued by therapy with the HDACi JNJ-26481585. Eur J Hum Genet 2013; 21(6): 643-52.
[http://dx.doi.org/10.1038/ejhg.2012.222] [PMID: 23073311]

[58]   Somers E, Lees RD, Hoban K, *et al.* Vascular Defects and Spinal Cord Hypoxia in Spinal Muscular Atrophy. Ann Neurol 2016; 79(2): 217-30.
[http://dx.doi.org/10.1002/ana.24549] [PMID: 26506088]

[59]   Deguise MO, De Repentigny Y, McFall E, Auclair N, Sad S, Kothary R. Immune dysregulation may contribute to disease pathogenesis in spinal muscular atrophy mice. Hum Mol Genet 2017; 26(4): 801-19.
[http://dx.doi.org/10.1093/hmg/ddw434] [PMID: 28108555]

[60]   Nery FC, Siranosian JJ, Rosales I, *et al.* Impaired kidney structure and function in spinal muscular atrophy. Neurol Genet 2019; 5(5)e353
[http://dx.doi.org/10.1212/NXG.0000000000000353] [PMID: 31517062]

[61]   Hensel N, Kubinski S, Claus P. The Need for SMN-Independent Treatments of Spinal Muscular Atrophy (SMA) to Complement SMN-Enhancing Drugs. Front Neurol 2020; 11: 45.
[http://dx.doi.org/10.3389/fneur.2020.00045] [PMID: 32117013]

[62]   Mendell JR, Al-Zaidy S, Shell R, *et al.* Single-Dose Gene-Replacement Therapy for Spinal Muscular Atrophy. N Engl J Med 2017; 377(18): 1713-22.
[http://dx.doi.org/10.1056/NEJMoa1706198] [PMID: 29091557]

[63]   Finkel RS, Mercuri E, Darras BT, *et al.* Nusinersen *versus* Sham Control in Infantile-Onset Spinal Muscular Atrophy. N Engl J Med 2017; 377(18): 1723-32.
[http://dx.doi.org/10.1056/NEJMoa1702752] [PMID: 29091570]

[64]   Tsai LK. Therapy development for spinal muscular atrophy in SMN independent targets. Neural Plast 2012; 2012456478
[http://dx.doi.org/10.1155/2012/456478] [PMID: 22701806]

[65]   Wadman RI, van der Pol WL, Bosboom WM, *et al.* Drug treatment for spinal muscular atrophy types II and III. Cochrane Database Syst Rev 2020; 1CD006282
[http://dx.doi.org/10.1002/14651858.CD006282.pub5] [PMID: 32006461]

[66]   Perego MGL, Galli N, Nizzardo M, *et al.* Current understanding of and emerging treatment options for spinal muscular atrophy with respiratory distress type 1 (SMARD1). Cell Mol Life Sci 2020; 77(17): 3351-67.
[http://dx.doi.org/10.1007/s00018-020-03492-0] [PMID: 32123965]

[67]   Lunke S, El-Osta A. Applicability of histone deacetylase inhibition for the treatment of spinal muscular atrophy. Neurotherapeutics 2013; 10(4): 677-87.
[http://dx.doi.org/10.1007/s13311-013-0209-2] [PMID: 23996601]

[68]   Wadman RI, van der Pol WL, Bosboom WM, *et al.* Drug treatment for spinal muscular atrophy type I. Cochrane Database Syst Rev 2019; 12CD006281
[http://dx.doi.org/10.1002/14651858.CD006281.pub5] [PMID: 31825542]

[69]   Mohseni J, Zabidi-Hussin ZA, Sasongko TH. Histone deacetylase inhibitors as potential treatment for spinal muscular atrophy. Genet Mol Biol 2013; 36(3): 299-307.
[http://dx.doi.org/10.1590/S1415-47572013000300001] [PMID: 24130434]

[70]   Calder AN, Androphy EJ, Hodgetts KJ. Small Molecules in Development for the Treatment of Spinal Muscular Atrophy. J Med Chem 2016; 59(22): 10067-83.
[http://dx.doi.org/10.1021/acs.jmedchem.6b00670] [PMID: 27490705]

[71]   Strahl BD, Allis CD. The language of covalent histone modifications. Nature 2000; 403(6765): 41-5.
[http://dx.doi.org/10.1038/47412] [PMID: 10638745]

[72]   Grzeschik SM, Ganta M, Prior TW, Heavlin WD, Wang CH. Hydroxyurea enhances SMN2 gene expression in spinal muscular atrophy cells. Ann Neurol 2005; 58(2): 194-202.
[http://dx.doi.org/10.1002/ana.20548] [PMID: 16049920]

[73]   Liang WC, Yuo CY, Chang JG, *et al.* The effect of hydroxyurea in spinal muscular atrophy cells and patients. J Neurol Sci 2008; 268(1-2): 87-94.
[http://dx.doi.org/10.1016/j.jns.2007.11.012] [PMID: 18166199]

[74]   Chen TH, Chang JG, Yang YH, *et al.* Randomized, double-blind, placebo-controlled trial of

hydroxyurea in spinal muscular atrophy. Neurology 2010; 75(24): 2190-7.
[http://dx.doi.org/10.1212/WNL.0b013e3182020332] [PMID: 21172842]

[75]   Angelozzi C, Borgo F, Tiziano FD, Martella A, Neri G, Brahe C. Salbutamol increases SMN mRNA and protein levels in spinal muscular atrophy cells. J Med Genet 2008; 45(1): 29-31.
[http://dx.doi.org/10.1136/jmg.2007.051177] [PMID: 17932121]

[76]   Kinali M, Mercuri E, Main M, *et al.* Pilot trial of albuterol in spinal muscular atrophy. Neurology 2002; 59(4): 609-10.
[http://dx.doi.org/10.1212/WNL.59.4.609] [PMID: 12196659]

[77]   Pane M, Staccioli S, Messina S, *et al.* Daily salbutamol in young patients with SMA type II. Neuromuscul Disord 2008; 18(7): 536-40.
[http://dx.doi.org/10.1016/j.nmd.2008.05.004] [PMID: 18579379]

[78]   Chen TH, Yang YH, Mai HH, *et al.* Reliability and validity of outcome measures of in-hospital and at-home visits in a randomized, double-blind, placebo-controlled trial for spinal muscular atrophy. J Child Neurol 2014; 29(12): 1680-4.
[http://dx.doi.org/10.1177/0883073813506935] [PMID: 24163397]

[79]   Singh NN, Shishimorova M, Cao LC, Gangwani L, Singh RN. A short antisense oligonucleotide masking a unique intronic motif prevents skipping of a critical exon in spinal muscular atrophy. RNA Biol 2009; 6(3): 341-50.
[http://dx.doi.org/10.4161/rna.6.3.8723] [PMID: 19430205]

[80]   Hua Y, Vickers TA, Okunola HL, Bennett CF, Krainer AR. Antisense masking of an hnRNP A1/A2 intronic splicing silencer corrects SMN2 splicing in transgenic mice. Am J Hum Genet 2008; 82(4): 834-48.
[http://dx.doi.org/10.1016/j.ajhg.2008.01.014] [PMID: 18371932]

[81]   Williams JH, Schray RC, Patterson CA, Ayitey SO, Tallent MK, Lutz GJ. Oligonucleotide-mediated survival of motor neuron protein expression in CNS improves phenotype in a mouse model of spinal muscular atrophy. J Neurosci 2009; 29(24): 7633-8.
[http://dx.doi.org/10.1523/JNEUROSCI.0950-09.2009] [PMID: 19535574]

[82]   Baughan TD, Dickson A, Osman EY, Lorson CL. Delivery of bifunctional RNAs that target an intronic repressor and increase SMN levels in an animal model of spinal muscular atrophy. Hum Mol Genet 2009; 18(9): 1600-11.
[http://dx.doi.org/10.1093/hmg/ddp076] [PMID: 19228773]

[83]   Porensky PN, Mitrpant C, McGovern VL, *et al.* A single administration of morpholino antisense oligomer rescues spinal muscular atrophy in mouse. Hum Mol Genet 2012; 21(7): 1625-38.
[http://dx.doi.org/10.1093/hmg/ddr600] [PMID: 22186025]

[84]   Chiriboga CA, Swoboda KJ, Darras BT, *et al.* Results from a phase 1 study of nusinersen (ISIS-SMN(Rx)) in children with spinal muscular atrophy. Neurology 2016; 86(10): 890-7.
[http://dx.doi.org/10.1212/WNL.0000000000002445] [PMID: 26865511]

[85]   Finkel RS, Chiriboga CA, Vajsar J, *et al.* Treatment of infantile-onset spinal muscular atrophy with nusinersen: a phase 2, open-label, dose-escalation study. Lancet 2016; 388(10063): 3017-26.
[http://dx.doi.org/10.1016/S0140-6736(16)31408-8] [PMID: 27939059]

[86]   Mercuri E, Darras BT, Chiriboga CA, *et al.* Nusinersen *versus* Sham Control in Later-Onset Spinal Muscular Atrophy. N Engl J Med 2018; 378(7): 625-35.
[http://dx.doi.org/10.1056/NEJMoa1710504] [PMID: 29443664]

[87]   Kariya S, Obis T, Garone C, *et al.* Requirement of enhanced Survival Motoneuron protein imposed during neuromuscular junction maturation. J Clin Invest 2014; 124(2): 785-800.
[http://dx.doi.org/10.1172/JCI72017] [PMID: 24463453]

[88]   De Vivo DC, Bertini E, Swoboda KJ, *et al.* Nusinersen initiated in infants during the presymptomatic stage of spinal muscular atrophy: Interim efficacy and safety results from the Phase 2 NURTURE

study. Neuromuscul Disord 2019; 29(11): 842-56.
[http://dx.doi.org/10.1016/j.nmd.2019.09.007] [PMID: 31704158]

[89] Dangouloff T, Burghes A, Tizzano EF, Servais L, Group NSS. 244th ENMC international workshop: Newborn screening in spinal muscular atrophy May 10-12, 2019, Hoofdorp, The Netherlands. Neuromuscul Disord 2020; 30(1): 93-103.
[http://dx.doi.org/10.1016/j.nmd.2019.11.002] [PMID: 31882184]

[90] Kariyawasam DST, Russell JS, Wiley V, Alexander IE, Farrar MA. The implementation of newborn screening for spinal muscular atrophy: the Australian experience. Genet Med 2020; 22(3): 557-65.
[http://dx.doi.org/10.1038/s41436-019-0673-0] [PMID: 31607747]

[91] Gidaro T, Servais L. Nusinersen treatment of spinal muscular atrophy: current knowledge and existing gaps. Dev Med Child Neurol 2018.
[PMID: 30221755]

[92] Talbot K, Tizzano EF. The clinical landscape for SMA in a new therapeutic era. Gene Ther 2017; 24(9): 529-33.
[http://dx.doi.org/10.1038/gt.2017.52] [PMID: 28644430]

[93] Messina S, Pane M, Sansone V, *et al.* Expanded access program with Nusinersen in SMA type I in Italy: Strengths and pitfalls of a successful experience. Neuromuscul Disord 2017; 27(12): 1084-6.
[http://dx.doi.org/10.1016/j.nmd.2017.09.006] [PMID: 29132728]

[94] Ramdas S, Servais L. New treatments in spinal muscular atrophy: an overview of currently available data. Expert Opin Pharmacother 2020; 21(3): 307-15.
[http://dx.doi.org/10.1080/14656566.2019.1704732] [PMID: 31973611]

[95] Nash LA, Burns JK, Chardon JW, Kothary R, Parks RJ. Spinal Muscular Atrophy: More than a Disease of Motor Neurons? Curr Mol Med 2016; 16(9): 779-92.
[http://dx.doi.org/10.2174/1566524016666161128113338] [PMID: 27894243]

[96] Kim JK, Jha NN, Feng Z, *et al.* Muscle-specific SMN reduction reveals motor neuron-independent disease in spinal muscular atrophy models. J Clin Invest 2020; 130(3): 1271-87.
[http://dx.doi.org/10.1172/JCI131989] [PMID: 32039917]

[97] Hua Y, Sahashi K, Rigo F, *et al.* Peripheral SMN restoration is essential for long-term rescue of a severe spinal muscular atrophy mouse model. Nature 2011; 478(7367): 123-6.
[http://dx.doi.org/10.1038/nature10485] [PMID: 21979052]

[98] Hua Y, Liu YH, Sahashi K, Rigo F, Bennett CF, Krainer AR. Motor neuron cell-nonautonomous rescue of spinal muscular atrophy phenotypes in mild and severe transgenic mouse models. Genes Dev 2015; 29(3): 288-97.
[http://dx.doi.org/10.1101/gad.256644.114] [PMID: 25583329]

[99] Gray SJ, Woodard KT, Samulski RJ. Viral vectors and delivery strategies for CNS gene therapy. Ther Deliv 2010; 1(4): 517-34.
[http://dx.doi.org/10.4155/tde.10.50] [PMID: 22833965]

[100] Bowers WJ, Breakefield XO, Sena-Esteves M. Genetic therapy for the nervous system. Hum Mol Genet 2011; 20(R1): R28-41.
[http://dx.doi.org/10.1093/hmg/ddr110] [PMID: 21429918]

[101] Foust KD, Wang X, McGovern VL, *et al.* Rescue of the spinal muscular atrophy phenotype in a mouse model by early postnatal delivery of SMN. Nat Biotechnol 2010; 28(3): 271-4.
[http://dx.doi.org/10.1038/nbt.1610] [PMID: 20190738]

[102] Al-Zaidy SA, Mendell JR. From Clinical Trials to Clinical Practice: Practical Considerations for Gene Replacement Therapy in SMA Type 1. Pediatr Neurol 2019; 100: 3-11.
[http://dx.doi.org/10.1016/j.pediatrneurol.2019.06.007] [PMID: 31371124]

[103] Valori CF, Ning K, Wyles M, *et al.* Systemic delivery of scAAV9 expressing SMN prolongs survival in a model of spinal muscular atrophy. Sci Transl Med 2010; 2(35)35ra42

[http://dx.doi.org/10.1126/scitranslmed.3000830] [PMID: 20538619]

[104] Pattali R, Mou Y, Li XJ. AAV9 Vector: a Novel modality in gene therapy for spinal muscular atrophy. Gene Ther 2019; 26(7-8): 287-95.
[http://dx.doi.org/10.1038/s41434-019-0085-4] [PMID: 31243392]

[105] Foust KD, Nurre E, Montgomery CL, Hernandez A, Chan CM, Kaspar BK. Intravascular AAV9 preferentially targets neonatal neurons and adult astrocytes. Nat Biotechnol 2009; 27(1): 59-65.
[http://dx.doi.org/10.1038/nbt.1515] [PMID: 19098898]

[106] McCarty DM, Monahan PE, Samulski RJ. Self-complementary recombinant adeno-associated virus (scAAV) vectors promote efficient transduction independently of DNA synthesis. Gene Ther 2001; 8(16): 1248-54.
[http://dx.doi.org/10.1038/sj.gt.3301514] [PMID: 11509958]

[107] Lowes LP, Alfano LN, Arnold WD, *et al.* Impact of Age and Motor Function in a Phase 1/2A Study of Infants With SMA Type 1 Receiving Single-Dose Gene Replacement Therapy. Pediatr Neurol 2019; 98: 39-45.
[http://dx.doi.org/10.1016/j.pediatrneurol.2019.05.005] [PMID: 31277975]

[108] Day JW, Chiriboga CA, Crawford TO, *et al.* Onasemnogene Abeparvovec-xioi Gene-Replacement Therapy for Spinal Muscular Atrophy Type 1: Phase 3 Study (STR1VE) Update. Anaheim, CA 2019 CureSMA Annual Conference.

[109] Mendell JR, Shell R, Lehman R, *et al.* Gene-Replacement Therapy in Spinal Muscular Atrophy Type 1: Long-Term Follow-Up From the Onsemnogene Abeparvovec-xioi Phase 1/2a Clinical Trial. Anaheim, CA 2019 CureSMA Annual Conference.

[110] Novartis announces AVXS-101 intrathecal study update Novartis[cited 2019 Dec 16] https://www.novartis.com/news/media-releases/novartis-announces-avxs-101-intrathecal-study-update

[111] van der Ploeg AT. The Dilemma of Two Innovative Therapies for Spinal Muscular Atrophy. N Engl J Med 2017; 377(18): 1786-7.
[http://dx.doi.org/10.1056/NEJMe1712106] [PMID: 29091554]

[112] Pan X, Yue Y, Zhang K, *et al.* AAV-8 is more efficient than AAV-9 in transducing neonatal dog heart. Hum Gene Ther Methods 2015; 26(2): 54-61.
[http://dx.doi.org/10.1089/hgtb.2014.128] [PMID: 25763686]

[113] Hinderer C, Katz N, Buza EL, *et al.* Severe Toxicity in Nonhuman Primates and Piglets Following High-Dose Intravenous Administration of an Adeno-Associated Virus Vector Expressing Human SMN. Hum Gene Ther 2018; 29(3): 285-98.
[http://dx.doi.org/10.1089/hum.2018.015] [PMID: 29378426]

[114] Colella P, Ronzitti G, Mingozzi F. Emerging Issues in AAV-Mediated *In Vivo* Gene Therapy. Mol Ther Methods Clin Dev 2017; 8: 87-104.
[http://dx.doi.org/10.1016/j.omtm.2017.11.007] [PMID: 29326962]

[115] Palacino J, Swalley SE, Song C, *et al.* SMN2 splice modulators enhance U1-pre-mRNA association and rescue SMA mice. Nat Chem Biol 2015; 11(7): 511-7.
[http://dx.doi.org/10.1038/nchembio.1837] [PMID: 26030728]

[116] Kletzl H, Marquet A, Günther A, *et al.* The oral splicing modifier RG7800 increases full length survival of motor neuron 2 mRNA and survival of motor neuron protein: Results from trials in healthy adults and patients with spinal muscular atrophy. Neuromuscul Disord 2019; 29(1): 21-9.
[http://dx.doi.org/10.1016/j.nmd.2018.10.001] [PMID: 30553700]

[117] Ratni H, Ebeling M, Baird J, *et al.* Discovery of Risdiplam, a Selective Survival of Motor Neuron-2 (SMN2) Gene Splicing Modifier for the Treatment of Spinal Muscular Atrophy (SMA). J Med Chem 2018; 61(15): 6501-17.
[http://dx.doi.org/10.1021/acs.jmedchem.8b00741] [PMID: 30044619]

[118] Sturm S, Günther A, Jaber B, *et al.* A phase 1 healthy male volunteer single escalating dose study of

the pharmacokinetics and pharmacodynamics of risdiplam (RG7916, RO7034067), a SMN2 splicing modifier. Br J Clin Pharmacol 2019; 85(1): 181-93.
[http://dx.doi.org/10.1111/bcp.13786] [PMID: 30302786]

[119]   Seabrook T, Baranello G, Servais L, *et al.* FIREFISH part 1: early clinical results following an increase of SMN protein in infants with type 1 spinal muscular atrophy (SMA) treated with Risdiplam (RG7916). Communication presented at MDA Clinical & Scientific Conference; April 13-17, 2019; Orlando, FL, USA

[120]   Mercuri E, Baranello G, Kirschner J, *et al.* Update from SUNFISH Part 1: safety, tolerability and PK/PD from the dose-finding study, including exploratory efficacy data, in patients with type 2 or 3 spinal muscular atrophy (SMA) treated with risdiplam (RG7916). Communication presented at American Academy of Neurology 2019-71st Annual Meeting; May 4-10, 2019, Philadelphia, PA, USA.

[121]   Roche's risdiplam meets primary endpoint in pivotal SUNFISH trial in people with type 2 or 3 spinal muscular atrophy Roche Available online https://www.roche.com/media/releases/med-cor-2019-11-11.html(accessed on 12 May 2019) (accessed on 12 May 2019).

[122]   Cheung AK, Hurley B, Kerrigan R, *et al.* Discovery of Small Molecule Splicing Modulators of Survival Motor Neuron-2 (SMN2) for the Treatment of Spinal Muscular Atrophy (SMA). J Med Chem 2018; 61(24): 11021-36.
[http://dx.doi.org/10.1021/acs.jmedchem.8b01291] [PMID: 30407821]

[123]   Jevtic S, Carr D, Dobrzycka-Ambrozevicz A, *et al.* Branaplam in Type 1 spinal muscular atrophy: second part of a phase I/II Study. Communication presented at 23rd SMA Researcher Meeting, Cure SMA; June 28-30, 2019; Anaheim, CA, USA.

[124]   Farooq F, Abadía-Molina F, MacKenzie D, *et al.* Celecoxib increases SMN and survival in a severe spinal muscular atrophy mouse model *via* p38 pathway activation. Hum Mol Genet 2013; 22(17): 3415-24.
[http://dx.doi.org/10.1093/hmg/ddt191] [PMID: 23656793]

[125]   Jarecki J, Chen X, Bernardino A, *et al.* Diverse small-molecule modulators of SMN expression found by high-throughput compound screening: early leads towards a therapeutic for spinal muscular atrophy. Hum Mol Genet 2005; 14(14): 2003-18.
[http://dx.doi.org/10.1093/hmg/ddi205] [PMID: 15944201]

[126]   Gogliotti RG, Cardona H, Singh J, *et al.* The DcpS inhibitor RG3039 improves survival, function and motor unit pathologies in two SMA mouse models. Hum Mol Genet 2013; 22(20): 4084-101.
[http://dx.doi.org/10.1093/hmg/ddt258] [PMID: 23736298]

[127]   Jędrzejowska M, Kostera-Pruszczyk A. Spinal muscular atrophy - new therapies, new challenges. Neurol Neurochir Pol 2020; 54(1): 8-13.
[http://dx.doi.org/10.5603/PJNNS.a2019.0068] [PMID: 31922583]

[128]   Van Meerbeke J, Gibbs R, Plasterer H, *et al.* The Therapeutic Effects of RG3039 in Severe Spinal Muscular Atrophy Mice and Normal Human Volunteers (S25.003). Neurology 2012; 78: 003. s25

[129]   Heier CR, DiDonato CJ. Translational readthrough by the aminoglycoside geneticin (G418) modulates SMN stability *in vitro* and improves motor function in SMA mice *in vivo.* Hum Mol Genet 2009; 18(7): 1310-22.
[http://dx.doi.org/10.1093/hmg/ddp030] [PMID: 19150990]

[130]   Cobb MS, Rose FF, Rindt H, *et al.* Development and characterization of an SMN2-based intermediate mouse model of Spinal Muscular Atrophy. Hum Mol Genet 2013; 22(9): 1843-55.
[http://dx.doi.org/10.1093/hmg/ddt037] [PMID: 23390132]

[131]   Greif H, Rosin-Arbesfeld R, Megiddo D. a read-through repurposed drug, shows proof of efficacy in SMA treatment. 2015.

[132]   Kwon DY, Motley WW, Fischbeck KH, Burnett BG. Increasing expression and decreasing

degradation of SMN ameliorate the spinal muscular atrophy phenotype in mice. Hum Mol Genet 2011; 20(18): 3667-77.
[http://dx.doi.org/10.1093/hmg/ddr288] [PMID: 21693563]

[133] Kaifer KA, Villalón E, Osman EY, *et al.* Plastin-3 extends survival and reduces severity in mouse models of spinal muscular atrophy. JCI Insight 2017; 2(5)e89970
[http://dx.doi.org/10.1172/jci.insight.89970] [PMID: 28289706]

[134] Sumner CJ, Crawford TO. Two breakthrough gene-targeted treatments for spinal muscular atrophy: challenges remain. J Clin Invest 2018; 128(8): 3219-27.
[http://dx.doi.org/10.1172/JCI121658] [PMID: 29985170]

[135] Bordet T, Buisson B, Michaud M, *et al.* Identification and characterization of cholest-4-en-3-one, oxime (TRO19622), a novel drug candidate for amyotrophic lateral sclerosis. J Pharmacol Exp Ther 2007; 322(2): 709-20.
[http://dx.doi.org/10.1124/jpet.107.123000] [PMID: 17496168]

[136] Bertini E, Dessaud E, Mercuri E, *et al.* Safety and efficacy of olesoxime in patients with type 2 or non-ambulatory type 3 spinal muscular atrophy: a randomised, double-blind, placebo-controlled phase 2 trial. Lancet Neurol 2017; 16(7): 513-22.
[http://dx.doi.org/10.1016/S1474-4422(17)30085-6] [PMID: 28460889]

[137] Haddad H, Cifuentes-Diaz C, Miroglio A, Roblot N, Joshi V, Melki J. Riluzole attenuates spinal muscular atrophy disease progression in a mouse model. Muscle Nerve 2003; 28(4): 432-7.
[http://dx.doi.org/10.1002/mus.10455] [PMID: 14506714]

[138] Merlini L, Solari A, Vita G, *et al.* Role of gabapentin in spinal muscular atrophy: results of a multicenter, randomized Italian study. J Child Neurol 2003; 18(8): 537-41.
[http://dx.doi.org/10.1177/08830738030180080501] [PMID: 13677579]

[139] Pirruccello-Straub M, Jackson J, Wawersik S, *et al.* Blocking extracellular activation of myostatin as a strategy for treating muscle wasting. Sci Rep 2018; 8(1): 2292.
[http://dx.doi.org/10.1038/s41598-018-20524-9] [PMID: 29396542]

[140] Feng Z, Ling KK, Zhao X, *et al.* Pharmacologically induced mouse model of adult spinal muscular atrophy to evaluate effectiveness of therapeutics after disease onset. Hum Mol Genet 2016; 25(5): 964-75.
[http://dx.doi.org/10.1093/hmg/ddv629] [PMID: 26758873]

[141] Liu M, Hammers DW, Barton ER, Sweeney HL. Activin Receptor Type IIB Inhibition Improves Muscle Phenotype and Function in a Mouse Model of Spinal Muscular Atrophy. PLoS One 2016; 11(11)e0166803
[http://dx.doi.org/10.1371/journal.pone.0166803] [PMID: 27870893]

[142] R&D Pipeline: ALG-801, AliveGen Available online http://www.alivegen.com/r-d-pipeline (accessed on 12 May 2020)

[143] Long KK, O'Shea KM, Khairallah RJ, *et al.* Specific inhibition of myostatin activation is beneficial in mouse models of SMA therapy. Hum Mol Genet 2019; 28(7): 1076-89.
[http://dx.doi.org/10.1093/hmg/ddy382] [PMID: 30481286]

[144] Chyung Y. Interim Results from a Phase 1 Study of SRK-015, a Fully Human Monoclonal Antibody that Inhibits Myostatin Activation. Communication presented at 23rd SMA researcher meeting, Cure SMA; June 28-30, 2019; Anaheim, CA, USA.

[145] Hwee DT, Kennedy AR, Hartman JJ, *et al.* The small-molecule fast skeletal troponin activator, CK-2127107, improves exercise tolerance in a rat model of heart failure. J Pharmacol Exp Ther 2015; 353(1): 159-68.
[http://dx.doi.org/10.1124/jpet.114.222224] [PMID: 25678535]

[146] Andrews JA, Miller TM, Vijayakumar V, *et al.* CK-2127107 amplifies skeletal muscle response to nerve activation in humans. Muscle Nerve 2018; 57(5): 729-34.

[http://dx.doi.org/10.1002/mus.26017] [PMID: 29150952]

[147] Day JW. Update of CY 5021: A Phase 2 Clinical Trial of Reldesemtiv, a Fast Skeletal Muscle Troponin Activator (FSTA), for the Potential Treatment of Spinal Muscular Atrophy. Communication presented at 22nd SMA Researcher Meeting, Cure SMA; June 14-16, 2018; Dallas, TX, USA.

[148] Wadman RI, Vrancken AF, van den Berg LH, van der Pol WL. Dysfunction of the neuromuscular junction in spinal muscular atrophy types 2 and 3. Neurology 2012; 79(20): 2050-5.
[http://dx.doi.org/10.1212/WNL.0b013e3182749eca] [PMID: 23115209]

[149] Stam M, Wadman RI, Wijngaarde CA, *et al.* Protocol for a phase II, monocentre, double-blind, placebo-controlled, cross-over trial to assess efficacy of pyridostigmine in patients with spinal muscular atrophy types 2-4 (SPACE trial). BMJ Open 2018; 8(7)e019932
[http://dx.doi.org/10.1136/bmjopen-2017-019932] [PMID: 30061431]

[150] Imlach WL, Beck ES, Choi BJ, Lotti F, Pellizzoni L, McCabe BD. SMN is required for sensory-motor circuit function in Drosophila. Cell 2012; 151(2): 427-39.
[http://dx.doi.org/10.1016/j.cell.2012.09.011] [PMID: 23063130]

[151] Pandolfi F, De Vita D, Bortolami M, *et al.* New pyridine derivatives as inhibitors of acetylcholinesterase and amyloid aggregation. Eur J Med Chem 2017; 141: 197-210.
[http://dx.doi.org/10.1016/j.ejmech.2017.09.022] [PMID: 29031067]

[152] Ebert AD, Yu J, Rose FF Jr, *et al.* Induced pluripotent stem cells from a spinal muscular atrophy patient. Nature 2009; 457(7227): 277-80.
[http://dx.doi.org/10.1038/nature07677] [PMID: 19098894]

[153] Corti S, Nizzardo M, Nardini M, *et al.* Neural stem cell transplantation can ameliorate the phenotype of a mouse model of spinal muscular atrophy. J Clin Invest 2008; 118(10): 3316-30.
[http://dx.doi.org/10.1172/JCI35432] [PMID: 18769634]

[154] Corti S, Nizzardo M, Nardini M, *et al.* Embryonic stem cell-derived neural stem cells improve spinal muscular atrophy phenotype in mice. Brain 2010; 133(Pt 2): 465-81.
[http://dx.doi.org/10.1093/brain/awp318] [PMID: 20032086]

[155] Poletti A, Fischbeck KH. Combinatorial treatment for spinal muscular atrophy: An Editorial for 'Combined treatment with the histone deacetylase inhibitor LBH589 and a splice-switch antisense oligonucleotide enhances SMN2 splicing and SMN expression in Spinal Muscular Atrophy cells' on page 264. J Neurochem 2020; 153(2): 146-9.
[http://dx.doi.org/10.1111/jnc.14974] [PMID: 32056234]

[156] Zhou H, Meng J, Malerba A, *et al.* Myostatin inhibition in combination with antisense oligonucleotide therapy improves outcomes in spinal muscular atrophy. J Cachexia Sarcopenia Muscle In press
[http://dx.doi.org/10.1002/jcsm.12542]

[157] Lee BH, Collins E, Lewis L, *et al.* Combination therapy with nusinersen and AVXS-101 in SMA type 1. Neurology 2019; 93(14): 640-1.
[http://dx.doi.org/10.1212/WNL.0000000000008207] [PMID: 31488615]

CHAPTER 2

Obesity Induced by the Neurological Drugs

Semiha Kurt[*], **Orhan Sumbul**, **Betul Cevik** and **Durdane Aksoy**
Tokat Gaziosmanpasa University, Faculty of Medicine, Department of Neurology, Tokat, Turkey

Abstract: Obesity is a serious health problem, especially in developed countries and poses an increasing danger. It is an important risk factor for some serious and chronic diseases, including hypertension, type II diabetes mellitus, coronary artery disease, stroke, and cancer. Obesity not only causes physical harm to patients but also leads to some common problems, such as low self-esteem, impaired psychosocial functioning, and low activity. Drug-induced weight gain and obesity may harm the patient instead of benefit. Treatment-induced weight gain is one of the important reasons for non-adherence to treatment. In particular, weight gain during adolescence is considered as an "unacceptable side effect" of drugs and causes drug discontinuation. Many drugs (antiepileptics, antidepressants, antipsychotics, *etc.*) used for the treatment of various neurological disorders are associated with weight gain. On the other hand, few drugs are associated with weight loss. In this chapter, the relationship between the drugs used in the treatment of various neurological disorders and weight change will be discussed.

Keywords: Antiepileptics, Antidepressants, Antipsychotics, Beta-blockers, Calcium channel blockers, Dopaminergic drugs, Glucocorticoids, Obesity, Neurological drugs, Serotonergic/ histaminergic agents, Weight gain.

INTRODUCTION

Weight gain has become a serious health problem, especially in developed countries in recent years. Overweight and obesity have become an epidemic public health problem, especially in children [1 - 4]. Obesity has tripled worldwide since 1975, as represented by the data from the World Health Organization (WHO) [5].

Weight stigma, another drawback for obese patients, is described as experiencing physical or verbal abuse secondary to the existence of obesity or overweight. Weight stigma causes negative consequences on individuals' health and emotions [6, 7].

[*] **Corresponding author Semiha Kurt**: Tokat Gaziosmanpaşa University, Faculty of Medicine Department of Neurology, Tokat, Turkey; Tel: +90 356 2125746/1260; Fax: +90 356 2133179; E-mail:gsemihakurt@hotmail.com

Atta-ur-Rahman & Zareen Amtul (Eds.)

Obesity is an important risk factor for some serious and chronic diseases, including hypertension, type II diabetes, coronary artery diseases, stroke, non-alcoholic steatohepatitis, and cancer [8]. Overweight and obesity are associated with increased mortality. Obesity not only causes physical harm to patients but also leads to some important problems, such as depression, low self-esteem, decreased psychosocial functionality, emotional and behavioral disorders, eating disorders, impaired body image, and low quality of life [9].

It is known that childhood obesity has important effects on both the physical and psychological health of children. Childhood obesity is associated with lower academic performance and lower quality of life [1, 4]. The studies have revealed the relationship of childhood obesity with neurological, metabolic, cardiovascular, orthopedic, liver, pulmonary, renal, dermatologic, and menstrual disorders. Childhood obesity has many health consequences, and three of the most common ones are sleep apnea, diabetes, and cardiovascular diseases [1, 4].

The drug-induced weight gain and obesity may cause harm to the patient rather than a benefit. Treatment-related weight gain is one of the important reasons for patients' non-adherence. Weight gain, especially during adolescence, is considered as an "unacceptable" side effect of drugs and causes drug discontinuation [10]. Many drugs (antiepileptics, antidepressants, antipsychotics, *etc.*) used for the treatment of various neurological diseases are associated with weight gain. On the other hand, few drugs are associated with weight loss [8].

In this section, the relationship between the drugs used in neurological diseases and weight changes will be discussed. While writing this chapter, clinical studies and meta-analyzes were especially used.

Antiepileptic Drugs (AEDs)

The patient's seizures and the type of epilepsy must be correctly classified to choose the appropriate antiepileptic drugs. The most important factors that play a role in drug selection can be summarized as effectiveness, absence of toxic effects or few side effects, interaction with other medication, comorbid medical conditions, age, gender, and cost based on a more realistic approach [11]. In addition, ease of use is an important factor for drugs, such as taking a single dose per day. For idiopathic generalized epilepsy (genetically mediated epilepsy), levetiracetam (LEV), lamotrigine (LTG), and valproate (VPA) are regarded as drugs selected by the experts; while zonisamide (ZNS) and topiramate (TPM) are regarded as commonly suitable or first-line drugs. For absence epilepsy, ethosuximide (ESM) is regarded as a selected drug, while LTG is regarded as a commonly suitable or first-line drug. ZNS is selected as a commonly suitable or first-line initial drug for myoclonic epilepsy [12]. For focal seizures with and without the loss of awareness (simple partial and complex partial seizures), the experts have evaluated LEV, LTG, and oxcarbazepine (OXC) as drugs of choice and commonly regarded carbamazepine (CBZ) as suitable or first-line [12]. Most of the new antiepileptics are used for therapy of focal epilepsy in addition to first-line drugs [12].

Antiepileptic drugs are the first-choice drugs in the treatment of neuropathic pain as well as epileptic seizures. Gabapentin (GBP), pregabalin (PGB), CBZ and OXC are among the top antiepileptic drugs used in the treatment of neuropathic pain [13]. Antiepileptics act by stabilizing neuronal membranes, increasing synaptic inhibition, or reducing synaptic excitation. CBZ and OXC cause voltage-gated sodium channel inactivation as well as reducing excitatory neurotransmitter release. GBP was originally designed as a GABA mimetic to freely cross the blood brain barrier. Now, it is assumed that it lacks GABAergic activity, and instead, it is connected in high affinity to alfa-2-delta-1 subunits of the voltage-gated calcium channels [14, 15]. PGB is a voltage-gated Ca channel modulator, reducing the excitatory neurotransmitter release. Pregabalin does not directly bind to GABA-A or GABA-B receptors and acts quickly. In recent years, it has become the first choice drug in neuropathic pain [16].

VPA and TPM are frequently used in the prophylactic treatment of migraine with similar mechanisms.

Few studies have been conducted on weight loss or weight gain in patients with epilepsy. In the study conducted on 8057 adults in the United States, 2.1% of patients had epilepsy, and it was found that even though their seizures were under control, they exercised less than others and were more prone to obesity (23.7% *versus* 34%) [17]. Similarly, another study conducted in Germany indicated that epileptics had higher body mass index (BMI) values and they did less exercise [18]. The frequency of obesity was higher in healthy epileptic patients compared to healthy controls [19]. There are very few epileptic genetic syndromes known to cause weight gain. Therefore, the three most important factors for explaining weight gain in epileptics are antiepileptic drugs, lifestyle, and concomitant depression [20].

AEDs may cause weight gain, weight loss or no weight changes (weight-neutral). The primary AEDs causing weight gain are VPA, PGB, GBP, CBZ, vigabatrin (VGB), ezogabine, and perampanel [21]. Those AEDs causing weight loss are TPM, felbamate, ZNS, rufinamide, and lacosamide [20, 21]. Weight-neutral drugs have been reported with phenytoin, OXC, LTG, LEV, and tiagabine [20].

Valproic Acid (VPA)

VPA is used in epilepsy, migraine prophylaxis, and bipolar disorders. In addition to obesity, it has been reported to cause endocrine diseases, such as hyperandrogenism, menstrual irregularities, anovulatory cycles, and polycystic ovary syndrome. This suggests that the underlying cause of the endocrine disorder is obesity-related insulin resistance and hyperinsulinemia [17]. VPA is also known to cause metabolic syndrome [20]. VPA is a GABA agonist and leads to an increase in membrane depolarization and may directly stimulate the hypothalamus, resulting in increased relish, hunger, and satisfaction for high-calorie drinks and energy consumption. VPA may directly stimulate pancreatic cells leading to hyperinsulinemia and adipocytes, further leading to hyperleptinemia. Insulin resistance has been proposed as the major mechanism of hyperleptinemia. Hyperinsulinemia leads to a decrease in blood glucose level, which stimulates the hypothalamus, leading to an increase in relish and afterwards weight gain and its results [20].

There are publications reporting weight gain ranging from 4 to 71% in different populations with VPA treatment [10]. Egger and Brett [22] reported weight gain in 44 out of 100 epileptic children treated with 30-50 mg / kg VPA daily. While weight gain did not occur at a low dose, it was evident at doses above 30 mg. There was no connection between epilepsy type or seizure control and weight gain.

Weight gain was reported in 20 out of 55 children who received VPA treatment. While weight gain was significantly associated with baseline body weight and BMI, no correlation was found with treatment onset age, duration of follow-up, gender, seizure type, etiology, and VPA dose [10].

The commonly accepted idea is that VPA is not a definitive clinical predictor of weight gain [20].

Neurohumoral factors likely to be responsible for VPA-induced weight gain are increased "GABA stimulation of the hypothalamus", "hyperinsulinism and insulin resistance", "hyperleptinemia and leptin resistance", "ghrelin and adiponectin", "glucagon-like peptide-1", "neuropeptide Y" and "galanin" [21].

Obesity-related fatty liver has also been reported in patients using VPA [20]. VPA can induce fatty acid binding protein 4 -disrupted lipid dysmetabolism without visible drug-induced liver injury [23].

Gabapentin (GBP)

The relationship between chronic high-dose GBP treatment and weight gain in 44 epileptic patients was investigated in an open study. The patients were followed up for more than 1 year, where 57% reported more than 5% increase in basal weight and 23% had an increment of more than 10%. GBP-related weight gain was not reported in double-blind placebo-controlled studies. However, all of these studies had less than 3 months of follow up time [17].

Felbamate

Felbamate is not used except for Lennox-Gastaut Syndrome due to the serious risk of toxicity. This drug is associated with weight loss in long-term clinical follow-up studies [17].

Lamotrigine (LTG)

LTG is considered to have no effect on weight. When the data of 32 clinical studies were retrospectively analyzed, weight change was reported as an average of 0.6 kg in men and 0.4 kg in women among 463 patients with epilepsy, using an average of 259 mg/ day LTG [24]. Similar findings were confirmed by a 32-week, double-blind study [25].

Pregabalin (PGB)

Weight gain has also been reported in PGB like gabapentin. In a double-blind placebo-controlled study in patients with epilepsy, weight gain was reported in 6% of the patients in the placebo group, 10% in the group receiving 150 mg/ day, and 12-14% in the group receiving 600 mg/ day. In the study conducted in patients suffering from neuropathic pain, the weight gain was observed in 3.1% of them in the placebo group (exceeding 7% of the basal weight) and in 11.4% in the treatment group [17]. A meta-analysis that included more than a hundred studies and more than 40 thousand patients treated with pregabalin revealed that 5/6 of the patients, for one year, conserved their baseline weight (no weight gain exceeding 7% of their baseline weight) while about 1/6 patients gained a weight exceeding 7% of baseline weight [26].

Dosage and duration of use are used as strong predictors for weight gain caused by PGB [21].

Topiramate (TPM)

TPM used for epilepsy and migraine prophylaxis is associated with weight loss [27]. Unlike other antiepileptic drugs, the weight loss effect of TPM has been demonstrated in double-blind placebo-controlled studies conducted with not only epileptic patients but also type 2 diabetic and nondiabetic obese patients and veterans [28, 29]. In an open study conducted with refractory epileptics [29], TPM was used at an average dose of 200 mg/ day for one year of treatment. Weight loss occurred in patients with a BMI of over 30. At least 5% of the initial weight decreased in 7 out of 8 patients with a BMI of over 30. The reduction in body weight was much more remarkable in obese patients than under-weight patients. One year after TPM treatment, obese people's food intake decreased by approximately 400 kcal/day; whereas, this reduction was around 20 kcal/ day in non-obese people. No significant changes in malabsorption or thyroid hormone and leptin levels were observed. Combined preparations of topiramate with phentermine are also used in the treatment of obesity [29, 30].

Zonisamide (ZNS)

Clinical trials in patients with epilepsy using zonisamide have consistently reported weight loss. In a randomized study conducted on 230 patients with resistant focal epilepsy, a significant weight loss was detected in patients using ZNS [17]. In a randomized, double-blind, placebo-controlled study in which 60 obese patients were using ZNS as a weight loss drug, ZNS group had a weight loss of average 5.9 kg and the placebo group had an average weight loss of 0.9 kg in the 16th week, while that in the 32nd week was 9.2 kg in ZNS group and 1.5 kg in the placebo group [17].

ZNS, used in the therapy of schizophrenic patients, also causes weight loss [31]. Weight loss in zonisamide treatment is associated with low serum leptin levels in overweight female epileptic patients [32]. Therefore, some countries have approved TPM and ZNS as anti-obesity medications [21].

Carbamazepine (CBZ)

Weight gain caused by water retention due to CBZ edema, hyponatremia, and hypoosmolarity in serum has been reported (8). Privetera *et al.* reported that while weight gain was detected in those using VPA, while there was no weight change in those using CBZ [33]. Again, in a randomized, open study conducted in 239 patients with newly diagnosed epilepsy that lasted for 24 weeks, only those using VPA had weight gain, while no weight change was observed in those using CBZ and LTG [17]. Some researchers have suggested that CBZ does not have a significant effect on weight [34].

Oxcarbazepine (OXC)

While most of the studies conducted in pediatric and adult populations have not reported a significant weight gain due to the use of OXC, there are studies stating that the use of OXC resulted in increased weight [35].

Vigabatrin (VGB)

Vigabatrin is an anticonvulsant that acts by increasing GABA levels in the brain. It is effective in some childhood epilepsy syndromes and focal epilepsy, especially infantile spasm. Its use is limited because it causes visual field defects. In the European monotherapy study comparing VGB and CBZ, VGB was better tolerated, and caused weight gain in 11% of patients, on the other hand, CBZ caused weight gain in 5% of patients [10]. A more recent open, long-term Canadian vigabatrin study revealed a weight gain of 3.7 ± 0.2 kg [10].

Levetiracetam (LEV)

Although it is generally accepted that levetiracetam has no effect on weight, Gelisse *et al.* reported a dramatic weight loss in 19 patients receiving LEV treatment [36]. Another study conducted with children and adolescents using different antiepileptics demonstrated that weight gain was observed at the lowest rate for LEV [37], while Pickrell *et al.* reported a significant weight gain [38].

Possible Causes of Antiepileptics Induced Weight Gains

The possible mechanisms of weight gain associated with antiepileptics have not yet been exactly clarified and drugs can lead to weight gain by different mechanisms. One of the possible mechanisms is that low blood glucose level affects the hypothalamus and stimulates eating. A low blood glucose level may be due to the race between them to bind drug and long-chain fatty acid to albumin. A long-chain fatty acid that cannot be connected to the albumin increases the insulin stimulation. An increase in insulin stimulation lowers serum glucose levels. Another possible explanation of the low blood level may be the low carnitine induced by the drug. This will decrease fatty acid metabolism and increase glucose consumption. The increased effect of drug-induced GABA-mediated neurotransmission can increase carbohydrate intake and reduce energy consumption. Antidiuretic hormone-like effect, norepinephrine, or serotonin-mediated effects are rarely blamed for weight gain. Unfortunately, most of the studies investigating the relationship between antiepileptics and weight gain have not considered the underlying mechanisms [10, 17].

Antipsychotics

The use of antipsychotics is required for neurological diseases such as Parkinson's disease (PD) and dementia. Dementia is a progressive disease accompanied by many cognitive impairments, but there is no impairment in consciousness level. It is a known fact that as the elderly population increases in the world, the rate of dementia increases. It is estimated that more than 50 million patients with dementia live all around the world. Patients suffering from Alzheimer's disease account for about 2/3 of all dementia patients worldwide [39].

Behavioral and psychological symptoms of dementia result in institutionalization, more cognitive impairment, worse quality of life, increased caregiver stress, and increased mortality [39]. Antipsychotic drugs should be used with caution as they are prone to extrapyramidal side effects in patients with dementia. It is more convenient to use the dose as half or two-thirds of the normal adult dose. Atypical antipsychotics are often preferred primarily in patients with dementia due to extrapyramidal side effects. Specifically, activation of 5-HT_{1A} receptors or inhibition of 5-HT_2, 5-HT_3, and 5-HT_6 receptors can relieve extrapyramidal side effects induced both by antipsychotics alone or by the combination of antipsychotic drugs with cholinesterase inhibitors or 5-HT reuptake inhibitors [40]. In their large meta-analysis, Ralph and Espinet reported that antipsychotic treatment is associated with an increased risk of mortality in patients with dementia [41]. The increased risk of mortality was also demonstrated in a cohort study [42].

Atypical antipsychotics are used in the treatment of patients suffering from Parkinson's disease due to visual hallucinations, delusions, elementary illusions, and nightmares accompanying the primary disease picture. Psychotic symptoms in Parkinson's disease are observed in up to 60% of the patients [43]. If there is no reason for infection, electrolyte imbalance is the most likely reason to explain why the current psychotic state is the iatrogenic caused by levodopa, dopamine agonists, amantadine, anticholinergics, and MAO-B inhibitors used in the treatment of Parkinson's disease. Psychotic symptoms are the most common reason for patients hospitalized in nursing homes. In this case, firstly, dopaminergic treatment is decreased with appropriate doses so as not to worsen the patient's motor symptoms. Psychotic symptoms persist in many patients despite this type of planned treatment. If psychotic symptoms persist, antipsychotic treatment is now required [43]. For psychosis of PD, the use of pimavanserin as the first-line treatment is approved by the FDA [43, 44]. Clozapine is also advisable but should be used with caution due to its serious side effect. Leukopenia is rare but seen in patients taking clozapine. Olanzapine and quetiapine should not be considered as first-line drugs for symptoms in Parkinson's disease [43]. Unfortunately, atypical antipsychotics, which are preferred due to the low amount of extrapyramidal side effects, cause a significant weight gain.

The use of atypical antipsychotic drugs gradually increases over time because of their effectiveness and fewer extrapyramidal side effects than the older generation typical antipsychotic drugs. The effects of atypical antipsychotic drugs on the gut microbiome are extremely interesting as their effects on metabolism and weight gain are known. Numerous studies have revealed that this weight gain induced by atypical antipsychotic drugs occurs as a result of the change of the microbiome composition. Notwithstanding, it is not yet clear how atypical antipsychotic drugs affect the microbiome [45].

Antipsychotic drugs can disturb lysosomal function by affecting cholesterol exchange; furthermore, antipsychotic drugs can prevent cholesterol biosynthesis by chemical similarity. The result of these molecular changes involves decreased high density lipoprotein and increased triglycerides and very low density lipoprotein that may translate into weight gain and be associated with metabolic disorders [46].

The FDA regards weight gain exceeding 7% of basal body weight as a significant result. In light of these data, clozapine, quetiapine, risperidone, olanzapine, and haloperidol are able to improve this significant increase in body weight [47].

Pimavanserin

The effect of pimavanserin, which is the only approved drug for psychosis of Parkinson's disease, on weight is not yet known. In the study conducted by Price *et al.* on rats, it was found that pimavanserin was effective in limiting weight gain due to high-fat food consumption only when used in high doses. Interestingly, the combined use of pimavanserin and lorcaserin was effective in decreasing both binge episodes and weight gain caused by high-fat food consumption [48]. In chronic schizophrenia patients, weight gain has been reported less with the combined use of antipsychotic drugs and pimavanserin [49]. Initial data have suggested that weight gain is less frequently observed with pimavanserin treatment.

Clozapine

The studies using clozapine have reported a high weight gain. There are studies reporting a weight gain ranging from 2.4 to 31.3 kg. Moreover, the weight gain induced by clozapine starts in the first 12 weeks of treatment and can prolong up to 4.5 years [50]. Some studies have reported that the rate of those who gained more than 7.5 kg of weight is 70% [50]. Among the 5 antipsychotics, including clozapine, olanzapine, risperidone, haloperidol, and sertindole, it has been found that clozapine and olanzapine both caused the most weight gain. Although some studies have reported that weight gain is greater in olanzapine, the general view is that it is higher in clozapine [51].

Quetiapine

It binds to D1, D2, 5-HT2a, 5-HT1a, and H1 receptors. Weight gain induced by quetiapine ranges from -1.5 to +4.1 kg [51]. Quetiapine is situated between risperidone and olanzapine in terms of its effect on weight gain. There was no significant weight gain in patients who switched from other antipsychotic medications to quetiapine [52]. There are studies reporting that quetiapine has a normalizing effect on weight (weight gain in underweight patients and weight loss in obese patients) [53].

Olanzapine

It affects many receptors, where D1, 5-HT2c, and H1 affinities are high. Controlled studies have proven that it increases weight gain. The rate of those who gain weight 7% or more as a result of the use of olanzapine is 31-90% [54]. Weight gain has been observed independent of the dose of olanzapine.

In patients taking any antipsychotic drug for the first time, weight gain is very important in the first 6 weeks because thereafter, patients do not lose weight [55]. Even 38 weeks after starting treatment with olanzapine, weight gain continues to increase [56].

Possible Causes of Weight Gain Caused by Antipsychotics

Various mechanisms are proposed regarding how antipsychotics cause weight gain.

Concerning the increase in food intake, atypical antipsychotics have been shown to modulate metabolic homeostasis in the hypothalamus, through their effects on neurotransmitter receptors such as dopamine (D2), serotonin (5-HT2c, 5-HT1b, 5-HT1a, 5-HT6), histamine (H1, H3), acetylcholine (M3), and adrenaline (alpha 2) [57].

Receptor affinity differences can be important in weight gain. Dopamine- related reward pathways are disturbed in patients treated with antipsychotic medicine and this disturbance may lead to changes in the ingestion of food and weight gain [58].

Serotonergic system; It is effective in the regulation of eating behavior and body weight. There are also data suggesting that serotonin (5-HT) plays a role in the regulation of leptin secretion. In particular, the 5-HT2C serotonin receptor has an important place in the regulation of eating. Feeding in rats decreases with 5-HT2C stimulation and increases with antagonist agents. Mice without 5-HT2C receptors eat more, get fat, respond to d-fenfluramine less, and are more likely to catch late-onset diabetes mellitus. Atypical antipsychotics are also thought to exert their effects on the 5-HT2C receptor [57 - 59].

The histaminergic system regulates leptin-related eating behavior through the hypothalamic histamine H1 receptor subtype. Food intake is suppressed by postsynaptic H1 receptor activation. It is known that as the H1 affinity increases, the sedation effect increases. A strong correlation was found between H1 receptor affinity and weight gain in antipsychotics [57, 59]. This information is supported by the fact that clozapine and olanzapine with the highest histaminergic activity are antipsychotics that cause the most weight gain, while tyioridazine and chlorpromazine have the same effect as typical antipsychotics. The blockage of the H1 receptor also increases appetite. Sedation is expected to increase weight gain by decreasing activity and basal metabolic rate [57, 59].

Atypical antipsychotics have a stimulatory effect on adrenergic α2 receptors. These receptors may affect weight gain [57].

Depending on the anticholinergic effect, people feel thirst and an increased appetite. Stimulation of muscarinic M3 receptors can cause weight gain [57].

Leptin is a cytokine derived from adipose cells and is proportional to the fat level in the body. It decreases nutrient intake, increases the thermogenic activity of the sympathetic nervous system, and forms a negative feedback ring with neuropeptides. Circulating leptin in humans is closely related to BMI, and the weight gain caused by atypical antipsychotics is also associated with leptin levels. Clozapine and olanzapine, which are the most weight-increasing antipsychotics, significantly increase serum leptin levels. However, it is still unknown if antipsychotic drugs cause leptin elevation through a direct mechanism or weight gain [57].

Epigenetic mechanisms are thought to be effective in obesity. CREB- regulated transcription coactivator 1 (CRTC1) gene has an important mission in the regulation of energy homeostasis. Remarkable methylation alterations were observed in three CRTC1 CpG regions in psychiatric patients with early and significant weight gain [60].

Antidepressants

Antidepressant drugs are frequently used agents in the treatment of headaches, especially tricyclics. There are common mechanisms such as inflammation and irregular hypothalamic function between headache and obesity. There are also publications on the reduction of pain frequency with diet, especially ketogenic diet, in obese patients with headache [61, 62]. In a meta-analysis conducted by Haynes *et al.*, with both longitudinal and cross-sectional studies, they stated that overweight perception was associated with both increased depressive symptoms and suicide risk [63]. There is a bidirectional relationship between depression and obesity [64].

In a population-based cohort study that was followed up for 10 years, patients using antidepressants had more than 5% weight gain compared to those who did not. The risk of weight gain actually increased during the 2nd and 3rd years of antidepressant treatment [65].

Tricyclic Antidepressants

Tricyclic antidepressants (TCAs) were used to treat depression in the past. But today, it is used more frequently in the treatment of neuropathic pain and migraine and tension-type headache than depression. The acute and chronic effects of TCAs on weight are generally well known [66]. TCAs, like amitriptyline and imipramine, cause more weight gain than other TCAs such as desipramine and nortriptyline. In a 2-year study conducted on 217 patients to evaluate weight gain associated with amitriptyline and mirtazapine, it was reported to be greater than 7% in the amitriptyline group and 22% in the mirtazapine group [66]. There are publications reporting an average weight gain of 3-4 kg with imipramine and 2 kg with amitriptyline [54]. In a study conducted using amitriptyline, nortriptyline, and paroxetin, weight gain detected in TCA users was found to be associated with serum levels of TNF p75 [67]. Among 1157 elderly patients who had been using antidepressants for at least 6 months, weight loss was not observed with TCAs, but was reported with selective serotonin reuptake inhibitors (SSRIs). Protriptyline is a TCA that inhibits small amounts of serotonin reuptake. Unlike other TCAs, it causes weight loss. Fewer headaches (86%) and a weight loss of 1.5 kg were detected in patients with chronic tension type headaches. It may be considered to replace the treatment with protriptyline in patients with headache who started to gain weight with TCAs [66].

Weight gain associated with TCAs may be related to histaminergic and adrenergic receptors, perhaps TNF levels. While activation of histamine receptors reduces hypothalamus-mediated food intake, some of the TCAs antagonize histamine receptors. Adrenergic receptors regulate eating behavior in the hypothalamus. TCAs can increase appetite in the synaptic range by causing an increase in norepinephrine [66].

Despite the publications reporting that TCAs increase weight gain in the early period, no relationship has been reported between TCA and weight gain in long-term follow-up studies. This suggests that TCAs do not increase weight in their long-term use [47].

Selective Serotonin Reuptake Inhibitors (SSRIs)

In addition to TCAs, SSRIs are also used successfully in tension headaches and migraine prophylaxis. Weight changes associated with SSRIs vary, depending on one of SSRIs and the duration of treatment. SSRIs, such as paroxetine and sertraline, can lead to weight gain compared to fluoxetine. A placebo-controlled study conducted with 832 patients using fluoxetine revealed that it was not associated with weight gain. In two studies, one of which lasted for 6 weeks and the other for 8 weeks, sertraline was reported to cause weight loss of 0.6 and 0.8 kg [66].

In more recent studies, SSRIs have been reported to cause weight loss in the short term, while weight gain in the long term. In a long-term study using fluoxetine, a weight gain of 2-2.5 kg was reported [54].

It is not surprising that SSRIs cause weight gain. In particular, the 5-HT receptor subtype is thought to be effective on appetite in the hypothalamus. Drugs that block the 5-HT receptor block the gene of this receptor in animals, thus increasing food intake and leading to insulin resistance and impaired glucose tolerance [66].

Selective Serotonin-Noradrenaline Reuptake Inhibitors (SNRIs)

Duloxetine and venlafaxine are antidepressants with both serotonin and noradrenaline reuptake inhibitors. Duloxetine and venlafaxine are the first-line medicines with strong advice based on evidence for all neuropathic pain cases [13].

They are effective in treating neuropathic pain and headache. It was also shown in a meta-analysis that SNRIs were effective in migraine preventive treatment [68]. In a short-term study using venlafaxine, 41 of 42 migraine patients stated to have weight loss [66]. There were patients who were excluded from another study due to loss of weight and appetite during duloxetine treatment [69]. However, in a 10-year follow-up study, venlafaxine and duloxetine users were reported to be at high risk for a weight gain of 5% [65].

Beta-Blockers

Beta-blockers were initially used in the treatment of hypertension and cardiac ischemia, and later in migraine prophylaxis. The most commonly used beta-blockers are propranolol, timolol, metoprolol, atenolol, and nadolol. Interestingly, how beta-blockers have prophylactic effects in migraine is not known exactly [66]. In chronic use, beta-blockers have been reported to be associated with weight gain in some patients. Several studies using beta-blockers for short-term migraine prophylaxis have not reported weight gain [66]. In an 8-week study comparing pizotifen and metoprolol in migraine prophylaxis, over 2 kg weight gain was reported in 53% of patients and only 6% of patients using metoprolol. In the long-term follow-up of 3800 patients who had a heart attack treated with propranolol, an average weight gain of 3 kg was reported 24 months later. In the meta-analysis of 8 controlled trials that lasted for at least 6 months using beta-blockers, weight gain increased by 3.4 kg more than the placebo group [66]. Weight gain induced by beta-blockers varies among studies. While some studies have stated that there is no weight gain, some others have reported otherwise [66]. Alpha-adrenergic receptors inhibit lipolysis; on the other hand, beta-adrenergic receptors stimulate lipolysis. Weight gain associated with chronic use of beta-blockers may be due to interactions of catecholamines with lipolysis. It is not clear whether or not there is a difference between non-selective beta-blockers (such as propranolol, nadolol) blocking both $\beta1$ and $\beta2$ receptors, and selective beta-blockers (such as metoprolol) blocking only $\beta1$ receptors in terms of weight gain. The use of beta-blockers can increase the development of type 2 diabetes and insulin resistance. It has been reported that the risk of developing type 2 diabetes increases by 28% in those who use beta-blockers among hypertensive patients compared to those who do not [70]. Reducing enzyme activity associated with lipid metabolism, influencing insulin secretion, and reducing peripheral blood flow may be mechanisms responsible for weight gain. Despite current metabolic risks, clinical studies have revealed beneficial effects of beta-blockers on mortality and morbidity in the treatment of hypertension, heart attack, and heart failure [70].

Beta-blockers are characteristically associated with weight gain during the first months of therapy, followed by a plateau. The weight gain induced by beta-blockers is mild and may not be clinically relevant [51].

Calcium Channel Blockers

Calcium channel blockers, such as verapamil, were originally used in the treatment of cardiac arrhythmia, but are now also used in migraine prophylaxis. The effectiveness of this group of drugs is not surprising in the migraine prophylaxis and cluster headaches. Because recent studies have demonstrated that mutation in P/Q calcium channel subtype is present in familial hemiplegic migraine [66]. Both verapamil and flunarizine are effective in preventing migraine. The effects of calcium channel blockers on weight may depend on their pharmacological effects except for the calcium channel. For example, flunarizine may act as a dopamine receptor antagonist, leading to weight gain. The relationship between flunarizine and weight gain has long been known. In the migraine prophylaxis study using flunarizine, 21% of the patients had an average weight gain of 4.3 kg at the end of the 4th month. In a double-blind study, flunarizine, which was used in migraine prophylaxis, caused an average weight gain of 4.5 kg in 29% of patients within 4 months [66]. In a large study, including 149 migraine patients, 23 out of 73 patients using flunarizine had an average weight gain of 1.9 kg within 5 months [65]. Another calcium channel blocker, verapamil, had no effect on weight. There are publications indicating that calcium channel blockers cause metabolic syndrome [70].

Serotonergic / Histaminergic Agents

Some drugs used in migraine prophylaxis, such as pizotifen and cyproheptadine, block serotonin and histamine. Chronic use of these drugs is closely associated with weight gain.

Pizotifen is a drug that has been used for many years in migraine prophylaxis. Blockade of 5HT2 and 5HT1C serotonin receptors, H1 histamine receptor, and muscarinic cholinergic receptors may be responsible for their side effects. Weight gain is the main reason that limits its use in migraine prophylaxis. In the first 12 weeks, weight gain of 4.1-5 kg has been reported with the use of pizotifen [66]. In a double-blind cross-study, 27 migraine patients had a weight gain of 4.1 kg within 2 months due to pizotifen [66]. In another double-blind crossover study, half of the migraine patients treated with pizotifen reported a weight gain of 2 - 10.5 kg within 8 weeks [66]. At least part of the weight gain due to pizotifene is associated with its antihistaminergic and anticholinergic effects. It is well known that these effects increase appetite and sedation.

Cyproheptadine is another drug that blocks both serotonin and histamine receptors and is used successfully in migraine prophylaxis. It is also used in anorexia and a few other weight loss diseases due to its appetite-enhancing feature [66].

Methysergide is a semi-synthetic ergot alkaloid derivative. It is not a common drug for migraine prophylaxis, as it can rarely cause fibrosis, which can be fatal in the retroperitoneal, lungs, or endocardium. Methysergide inhibits the release of histamine from mast cells by blocking serotonin receptors. In 500 patients with migraine and cluster headache, weight gain caused by methysergide was reported. It is not surprising that both antihistaminergic and serotonergic activity-related drugs lead to weight gain, as mentioned earlier [66].

Glucocorticoids

Glucocorticoids are used in many diseases that affect the immune system and cause inflammation. It is well known that glucocorticoids increase weight and blood pressure, if used for a long time. Glucocorticoids increase gluconeogenesis in the liver and inhibit insulin release from pancreatic cells, leading to weight gain, insulin resistance, and impaired glucose uptake [71]. There is evidence indicating that glucocorticoids regulate appetite, energy balance, and metabolic processes by increasing endocannabinoid signals both centrally and through peripheral pathways [72]. Weight loss caused by exercise, diet, and bariatric surgery is associated with decreased glucocorticoid secretion and function. It may also be associated with the improvement of insulin sensitivity and function of insulin sensitivity proteins [71].

An alternate-day dosing schedule for prednisone can reduce weight gain and even cause weight loss [51].

Dopaminergic Drugs

Parkinson's disease (PD) is the second most common neurodegenerative disease after Alzheimer's. Cardinal clinical symptoms of PD include bradykinesia, rigidity, tremor, and postural instability. In the treatment of Parkinson's disease, dopaminergic drugs are used to increase the reduced dopaminergic transition. For this purpose, the most frequently used and the most effective drugs are preparations containing levodopa. The second group of drugs used to increase dopaminergic transition is dopamine agonists. These drugs bind to dopamine receptors and mimic the effect of dopamine [73, 74].

There are publications reporting that both overweight and low weight are risk factors for PD [74, 75]. Nevertheless, a significant number of PD patients are underweight and generally lose weight during the course of the disease; whereas, some patients show an increase [76].

There are publications reporting that there is an inverse relationship between BMI and levodopa or the total dose of dopaminergic drugs in patients suffering from PD [76]. Patients receiving higher doses of levodopa have lower BMI values. As the dose of levodopa increases, the dyskinesias of the patients increases. As expected in the study of Bachmann *et al.*, patients using higher levodopa had more dyskinesias [76]. It is thought that the increase in dyskinesia may cause weight loss as it increases energy consumption. However, it is not fully understood how dopaminergic drugs affect weight.

Dopamine agonists, which cause much less dyskinesia, do not cause any significant change in BMI [77, 78]. Dopamine agonists can facilitate eating by increasing the patient's motor movements and increasing hand-mouth coordination but may cause nausea and decreased appetite. In the light of these findings, weight loss, as well as weight gain, have been reported with agonists. However, it is generally accepted that dopamine agonists have no effect on weight [77, 78].

Amantadine improves the symptoms of Parkinson's disease with an indirect dopaminergic effect. In the double-blind, placebo-controlled study conducted by Karen *et al.*, BMI value of patients who received olanzapine had an increase of 1.24 kg/ m^2 in the placebo group, while it had a decrease of 0.07 kg/ m^2 in the amantadine group [79].

Table 1. Treatment-related weight changes associated with neurological drugs.

Drugs	*Weight Effect*
Antiepileptic Drugs [20, 21]	
Carbamazepine	Gain
Ezogabine	Gain
Felbamate	Loss
Gabapentin	Gain
Lacosamide	Loss

(Table 1) cont.....

Drugs	Weight Effect
Lamotrigine	Neutral
Levetiracetam	Neutral
Oxcarbazepine	Neutral
Perampanel	Gain
Phenytoin	Neutral
Pregabalin	Gain
Rufinamide	Loss
Tiagabine	Neutral
Topiramate	Loss
Valproate	Gain
Vigabatrin	Gain
Zonisamide	Loss
Antipsychotics	
Clozapine [50, 51]	Gain (high)
Olanzapine [54-56]	Gain (high)
Pimavanserin [48, 49]	Gain (low)
Quetiapine [53]	Normalizing effect
Antidepressants	
Amitriptyline [54]	Gain (low)
Duloxetine [65, 66]	Short-term loss, long-term gain
Fluoxetine [54]	Short-term loss, long-term gain
Imipramine [54]	Gain (low)
Protriptyline [66]	Loss
Venlafaxine [65, 66]	Short-term loss, long-term gain
Beta-blockers *[51]*	Gain (low)
Calcium Channel Blockers	
Flunarizine [65, 66]	Gain (intermediate)
Verapamil [70]	Neutral
Serotonergic / histaminergic agents *[66]*	Gain
Glucocorticoids *[71, 72]*	Gain
Dopaminergic Drugs	
Amantadine [79]	Loss (low)
Dopamine agonists [77, 78]	Neutral
Levodopa [76]	Loss

CONCLUDING REMARKS

Overweight and obesity concern all areas of medicine as they negatively affect overall health. The first step in the treatment should be to weigh the patients each time to review their weight changes and calculate their BMI. Some patients may also need to measure the waist circumference. The possibility of weight change should be discussed with the patient before starting treatment. The effects of drugs used in neurological diseases on weight are summarized in Table **1**. Although it is difficult to differentiate the "normal" weight gain that can develop over time from iatrogenic obesity, it should be remembered that weight gain makes adherence to treatment difficult [1].

In case of weight gain or unwanted weight loss, special treatments should be considered. In the case of weight gain, diet and exercise are the first steps. In the second step, drugs that prevent weight gain can be considered. There are publications reporting that drugs such as topiramate, fluoxetine, and amantadine are useful in the treatment of obesity developing secondary to treatment [8]. However, there are publications indicating that these approaches are not effective in losing weight. In this case, changing the drug thought to be responsible for weight gain should be considered. In fact, if the effectiveness of drugs that do not cause weight gain in overweight or obese people is proven and they do not adversely affect the other comorbids of the patient, they may be preferred.

Phentermine HCl, orlistat, phentermine/topiramate ER, lorcaserin, naltrexone SR/bupropion SR, and liraglutide 3.0 mg are commonly used drugs in the treatment of obesity [80, 81]. There are data indicating that metformin facilitates weight loss in those using antipsychotic drugs [64]. Although diet and exercise are reported as first-line therapy in guidelines for drug-induced obesity [1], a recent meta-analysis reporting that lifestyle interventions (diet, exercise, or both) are "statistically significant but clinically insignificant" in patients with serious mental illnesses [82]. Weight gain in the first month after the onset of psychotropic drugs is a potent predictor of long-term weight gain [83]. Therefore, weight should be monitored before and shortly after initiating an antipsychotic drug treatment and an increase of 5% above basal weight after the first month should actuate doctors to reconsider therapy choices or to start weight controlling tactics [83].

Maybe in the future, predictive genetic testing for drug-induced weight gain would indicate a first-step towards individualized drugs addressing this dangerous and difficult iatrogenic disease [84].

CONSENT FOR PUBLICATION

Not applicable.

CONFLICT OF INTEREST

The author confirms that this chapter content has no conflict of interest.

ACKNOWLEDGEMENTS

Declared none.

REFERENCES

[1]   Sanyaolu A, Okorie C, Qi X, Locke J, Rehman S. Childhood and Adolescent Obesity in the United States: A Public Health Concern 2019.
[http://dx.doi.org/10.1177/2333794X19891305]

[2]   Chiavaroli V, Gibbins JD, Cutfield WS, Derraik JGB. Childhood obesity in New Zealand. World J Pediatr 2019; 15(4): 322-31.
[http://dx.doi.org/10.1007/s12519-019-00261-3] [PMID: 31079339]

[3]   Di Cesare M, Sorić M, Bovet P, *et al.* The epidemiological burden of obesity in childhood: a worldwide epidemic requiring urgent action. BMC Med 2019; 17(1): 212.
[http://dx.doi.org/10.1186/s12916-019-1449-8] [PMID: 31760948]

[4]   Lee EY, Yoon KH. Epidemic obesity in children and adolescents: risk factors and prevention. Front Med 2018; 12(6): 658-66.
[http://dx.doi.org/10.1007/s11684-018-0640-1] [PMID: 30280308]

[5]   Geneva: World Health Organisation 2020. https://www.who.int/news-room/fact-sheets/detail/obesi-y-and-overweight

[6]   Alimoradi Z, Golboni F, Griffiths MD, Broström A, Lin CY, Pakpour AH. Weight-related stigma and psychological distress: A systematic review and meta-analysis 2019.
[http://dx.doi.org/10.1016/j.clnu.2019.10.016]

[7]   Wu YK, Berry DC. Impact of weight stigma on physiological and psychological health outcomes for overweight and obese adults: A systematic review. J Adv Nurs 2018; 74(5): 1030-42.
[http://dx.doi.org/10.1111/jan.13511] [PMID: 29171076]

[8]   Verhaegen AA, Van Gaal LF. Drug-induced obesity and its metabolic consequences: a review with a focus on mechanisms and possible therapeutic options. J Endocrinol Invest 2017; 40(11): 1165-74.
[http://dx.doi.org/10.1007/s40618-017-0719-6] [PMID: 28660606]

[9]   Chu DT, Minh Nguyet NT, Nga VT, *et al.* An update on obesity: Mental consequences and psychological interventions. Diabetes Metab Syndr 2019; 13(1): 155-60.
[http://dx.doi.org/10.1016/j.dsx.2018.07.015] [PMID: 30641689]

[10]   Jallon P, Picard F. Bodyweight gain and anticonvulsants: a comparative review. Drug Saf 2001; 24(13): 969-78.
[http://dx.doi.org/10.2165/00002018-200124130-00004] [PMID: 11735653]

[11]   Schachter SC. Overview of the management of epilepsy in adults 2020.
https://www.uptodate.com/contents/overview-of-the-management-of-epilepsy-in-adults#H5

[12]   Shih JJ, Whitlock JB, Chimato N, Vargas E, Karceski SC, Frank RD. Epilepsy treatment in adults and adolescents: Expert opinion, 2016. Epilepsy Behav 2017; 69: 186-222.
[http://dx.doi.org/10.1016/j.yebeh.2016.11.018] [PMID: 28237319]

[13]   Szok D, Tajti J, Nyári A, Vécsei L. Therapeutic Approaches for Peripheral and Central Neuropathic Pain. Behav Neurol 2019; 20198685954
[http://dx.doi.org/10.1155/2019/8685954] [PMID: 31871494]

[14]   Sills GJ, Rogawski MA. Mechanisms of action of currently used antiseizure drugs. Neuropharmacology 2020; 168107966
[http://dx.doi.org/10.1016/j.neuropharm.2020.107966] [PMID: 32120063]

[15]   Yasaei R, Katta S, Saadabadi A. Gabapentin.StatPearls. Treasure Island, FL: StatPearls Publishing 2020.

[16]   Cross AL, Viswanath O, Sherman AL. Pregabalin. StatPearls. Treasure Island, FL: StatPearls Publishing 2020.

[17]   Ben-Menachem E. Weight issues for people with epilepsy—A review. Epilepsia 2007; 48 (Suppl. 9): 42-5.
[http://dx.doi.org/10.1111/j.1528-1167.2007.01402.x] [PMID: 18047602]

[18]   Kobau R, DiIorio CA, Price PH, *et al.* Prevalence of epilepsy and health status of adults with epilepsy in Georgia and Tennessee: Behavioral Risk Factor Surveillance System, 2002. Epilepsy Behav 2004; 5(3): 358-66.
[http://dx.doi.org/10.1016/j.yebeh.2004.02.007] [PMID: 15145306]

[19]   Daniels ZS, Nick TG, Liu C, Cassedy A, Glauser TA. Obesity is a common comorbidity for pediatric patients with untreated, newly diagnosed epilepsy. Neurology 2009; 73(9): 658-64.
[http://dx.doi.org/10.1212/WNL.0b013e3181ab2b11] [PMID: 19474413]

[20]   Hamed SA. Antiepileptic drugs influences on body weight in people with epilepsy. Expert Rev Clin Pharmacol 2015; 8(1): 103-14.
[http://dx.doi.org/10.1586/17512433.2015.991716] [PMID: 25487080]

[21]   Chukwu J, Delanty N, Webb D, Cavalleri GL. Weight change, genetics and antiepileptic drugs. Expert Rev Clin Pharmacol 2014; 7(1): 43-51.
[http://dx.doi.org/10.1586/17512433.2014.857599] [PMID: 24308788]

[22]   Egger J, Brett EM. Effects of sodium valproate in 100 children with special reference to weight. Br Med J (Clin Res Ed) 1981; 283(6291): 577-81.
[http://dx.doi.org/10.1136/bmj.283.6291.577] [PMID: 6790086]

[23]   Li R, Liang L, Wu X, Ma X, Su M. Valproate acid (VPA)-induced dysmetabolic function in clinical and animal studies. Clin Chim Acta 2017; 468: 1-4.
[http://dx.doi.org/10.1016/j.cca.2017.01.030] [PMID: 28161274]

[24]   Devinsky O, Vuong A, Hammer A, Barrett PS. Stable weight during lamotrigine therapy: a review of 32 studies. Neurology 2000; 54(4): 973-5.
[http://dx.doi.org/10.1212/WNL.54.4.973] [PMID: 10690996]

[25]   Biton V, Mirza W, Montouris G, Vuong A, Hammer AE, Barrett PS. Weight change associated with valproate and lamotrigine monotherapy in patients with epilepsy. Neurology 2001; 56(2): 172-7.
[http://dx.doi.org/10.1212/WNL.56.2.172] [PMID: 11160951]

[26]   Cabrera J, Emir B, Dills D, Murphy TK, Whalen E, Clair A. Characterizing and understanding body weight patterns in patients treated with pregabalin. Curr Med Res Opin 2012; 28(6): 1027-37.
[http://dx.doi.org/10.1185/03007995.2012.684044] [PMID: 22494020]

[27]   Khalil NY, AlRabiah HK, Al Rashoud SS, Bari A, Wani TA. Topiramate: Comprehensive profile. Profiles Drug Subst Excip Relat Methodol 2019; 44: 333-78.
[http://dx.doi.org/10.1016/bs.podrm.2018.11.005] [PMID: 31029222]

[28]   Kazerooni R, Lim J. Topiramate-Associated Weight Loss in a Veteran Population. Mil Med 2016; 181(3): 283-6.
[http://dx.doi.org/10.7205/MILMED-D-14-00636] [PMID: 26926755]

[29]   Antel J, Hebebrand J. Weight-reducing side effects of the antiepileptic agents topiramate and zonisamide. Handb Exp Pharmacol 2012; (209): 433-66.
[http://dx.doi.org/10.1007/978-3-642-24716-3_20] [PMID: 22249827]

[30]   Garvey WT, Ryan DH, Look M, *et al.* Two-year sustained weight loss and metabolic benefits with controlled-release phentermine/topiramate in obese and overweight adults (SEQUEL): a randomized, placebo-controlled, phase 3 extension study. Am J Clin Nutr 2012; 95(2): 297-308.
[http://dx.doi.org/10.3945/ajcn.111.024927] [PMID: 22158731]

[31]   Yang J, Lee MS, Joe SH, Jung IK, Kim SH. Zonisamide-induced weight loss in schizophrenia: case series. Clin Neuropharmacol 2010; 33(2): 104-6.
[http://dx.doi.org/10.1097/WNF.0b013e3181c848a0] [PMID: 19935403]

[32]   Kim DW, Yoo MW, Park KS. Low serum leptin level is associated with zonisamide-induced weight loss in overweight female epilepsy patients. Epilepsy Behav 2012; 23(4): 497-9.
[http://dx.doi.org/10.1016/j.yebeh.2011.11.024] [PMID: 22440324]

[33]   Privitera MD, Brodie MJ, Mattson RH, Chadwick DW, Neto W, Wang S. Topiramate, carbamazepine and valproate monotherapy: double-blind comparison in newly diagnosed epilepsy. Acta Neurol Scand 2003; 107(3): 165-75.
[http://dx.doi.org/10.1034/j.1600-0404.2003.00093.x] [PMID: 12614309]

[34]   Grootens KP, Meijer A, Hartong EG, *et al.* Weight changes associated with antiepileptic mood stabilizers in the treatment of bipolar disorder. Eur J Clin Pharmacol 2018; 74(11): 1485-9.
[http://dx.doi.org/10.1007/s00228-018-2517-2] [PMID: 30083876]

[35]   Garoufi A, Vartzelis G, Tsentidis C, *et al.* Weight gain in children on oxcarbazepine monotherapy. Epilepsy Res 2016; 122: 110-3.
[http://dx.doi.org/10.1016/j.eplepsyres.2016.03.004] [PMID: 27010568]

[36]   Gelisse P, Juntas-Morales R, Genton P, *et al.* Dramatic weight loss with levetiracetam. Epilepsia 2008; 49(2): 308-15.
[http://dx.doi.org/10.1111/j.1528-1167.2007.01273.x] [PMID: 17825078]

[37]   Egunsola O, Choonara I, Sammons HM, Whitehouse WP. Safety of antiepileptic drugs in children and young people: A prospective cohort study. Seizure 2018; 56: 20-5.
[http://dx.doi.org/10.1016/j.seizure.2018.01.018] [PMID: 29427834]

[38]   Pickrell WO, Lacey AS, Thomas RH, Smith PE, Rees MI. Weight change associated with antiepileptic drugs. J Neurol Neurosurg Psychiatry 2013; 84(7): 796-9.
[http://dx.doi.org/10.1136/jnnp-2012-303688] [PMID: 23236017]

[39]   Calsolaro V, Antognoli R, Okoye C, Monzani F. The Use of Antipsychotic Drugs for Treating Behavioral Symptoms in Alzheimer's Disease. Front Pharmacol 2019; 10: 1465.
[http://dx.doi.org/10.3389/fphar.2019.01465] [PMID: 31920655]

[40]   Ohno Y, Kunisawa N, Shimizu S. Antipsychotic Treatment of Behavioral and Psychological Symptoms of Dementia (BPSD): Management of Extrapyramidal Side Effects. Front Pharmacol 2019; 10: 1045.
[http://dx.doi.org/10.3389/fphar.2019.01045] [PMID: 31607910]

[41]   Ralph SJ, Espinet AJ. Increased All-Cause Mortality by Antipsychotic Drugs: Updated Review and Meta-Analysis in Dementia and General Mental Health Care. J Alzheimers Dis Rep 2018; 2(1): 1-26.
[http://dx.doi.org/10.3233/ADR-170042] [PMID: 30480245]

[42]   Schwertner E, Secnik J, Garcia-Ptacek S, *et al.* Antipsychotic Treatment Associated With Increased Mortality Risk in Patients With Dementia. A Registry-Based Observational Cohort Study. J Am Med Dir Assoc 2019; 20(3): 323-329.e2.
[http://dx.doi.org/10.1016/j.jamda.2018.12.019] [PMID: 30824220]

[43]   Zhang H, Wang L, Fan Y, *et al.* Atypical antipsychotics for Parkinson's disease psychosis: a systematic review and meta-analysis. Neuropsychiatr Dis Treat 2019; 15: 2137-49.

[http://dx.doi.org/10.2147/NDT.S201029] [PMID: 31551655]

[44]   Cummings J, Ritter A, Rothenberg K. Advances in Management of Neuropsychiatric Syndromes in Neurodegenerative Diseases. Curr Psychiatry Rep 2019; 21(8): 79.
[http://dx.doi.org/10.1007/s11920-019-1058-4] [PMID: 31392434]

[45]   Bretler T, Weisberg H, Koren O, Neuman H. The effects of antipsychotic medications on microbiome and weight gain in children and adolescents. BMC Med 2019; 17(1): 112.
[http://dx.doi.org/10.1186/s12916-019-1346-1] [PMID: 31215494]

[46]   Vantaggiato C, Panzeri E, Citterio A, Orso G, Pozzi M. Antipsychotics Promote Metabolic Disorders Disrupting Cellular Lipid Metabolism and Trafficking. Trends Endocrinol Metab 2019; 30(3): 189-210.
[http://dx.doi.org/10.1016/j.tem.2019.01.003] [PMID: 30718115]

[47]   Alonso-Pedrero L, Bes-Rastrollo M, Marti A. Effects of antidepressant and antipsychotic use on weight gain: A systematic review. Obes Rev 2019; 20(12): 1680-90.
[http://dx.doi.org/10.1111/obr.12934] [PMID: 31524318]

[48]   Price AE, Brehm VD, Hommel JD, Anastasio NC, Cunningham KA. Pimavanserin and Lorcaserin Attenuate Measures of Binge Eating in Male Sprague-Dawley Rats. Front Pharmacol 2018; 9: 1424.
[http://dx.doi.org/10.3389/fphar.2018.01424] [PMID: 30581386]

[49]   Meltzer HY, Elkis H, Vanover K, et al. Pimavanserin, a selective serotonin (5-HT)2A-inverse agonist, enhances the efficacy and safety of risperidone, 2mg/day, but does not enhance efficacy of haloperidol, 2mg/day: comparison with reference dose risperidone, 6mg/day. Schizophr Res 2012; 141(2-3): 144-52.
[http://dx.doi.org/10.1016/j.schres.2012.07.029] [PMID: 22954754]

[50]   Schwartz TL, Nihalani N, Jindal S, Virk S, Jones N. Psychiatric medication-induced obesity: a review. Obes Rev 2004; 5(2): 115-21.
[http://dx.doi.org/10.1111/j.1467-789X.2004.00139.x] [PMID: 15086865]

[51]   Wharton S, Raiber L, Serodio KJ, Lee J, Christensen RA. Medications that cause weight gain and alternatives in Canada: a narrative review. Diabetes Metab Syndr Obes 2018; 11: 427-38.
[http://dx.doi.org/10.2147/DMSO.S171365] [PMID: 30174450]

[52]   Hashimoto N, Toyomaki A, Honda M, et al. Long-term efficacy and tolerability of quetiapine in patients with schizophrenia who switched from other antipsychotics because of inadequate therapeutic response-a prospective open-label study. Ann Gen Psychiatry 2015; 14(1): 1.
[http://dx.doi.org/10.1186/s12991-014-0039-6] [PMID: 25632293]

[53]   Brecher M, Rak IW, Melvin K, Jones AM. The long-term effect of quetiapine (Seroquel TM) monotherapy on weight in patients with schizophrenia. Int J Psychiatry Clin Pract 2000; 4(4): 287-91.
[http://dx.doi.org/10.1080/13651500050517849] [PMID: 24926579]

[54]   Nihalani N, Schwartz TL, Siddiqui UA, Megna JL. Obesity and psychotropics. CNS Neurosci Ther 2012; 18(1): 57-63.
[http://dx.doi.org/10.1111/j.1755-5949.2011.00232.x] [PMID: 22070396]

[55]   Bak M, Fransen A, Janssen J, van Os J, Drukker M. Almost all antipsychotics result in weight gain: a meta-analysis. PLoS One 2014; 9(4)e94112
[http://dx.doi.org/10.1371/journal.pone.0094112] [PMID: 24763306]

[56]   Barton BB, Segger F, Fischer K, Obermeier M, Musil R. Update on weight-gain caused by antipsychotics: a systematic review and meta-analysis. Expert Opin Drug Saf 2020; 19(3): 295-314.
[http://dx.doi.org/10.1080/14740338.2020.1713091] [PMID: 31952459]

[57]   Endomba FT, Tankeu AT, Nkeck JR, Tochie JN. Leptin and psychiatric illnesses: does leptin play a role in antipsychotic-induced weight gain? Lipids Health Dis 2020; 19(1): 22.
[http://dx.doi.org/10.1186/s12944-020-01203-z] [PMID: 32033608]

[58]   Kaar SJ, Natesan S, McCutcheon R, Howes OD. Antipsychotics: Mechanisms underlying clinical

response and side-effects and novel treatment approaches based on pathophysiology. Neuropharmacology 2020; 172107704
[http://dx.doi.org/10.1016/j.neuropharm.2019.107704] [PMID: 31299229]

[59]   Marteene W, Winckel K, Hollingworth S, *et al.* Strategies to counter antipsychotic-associated weight gain in patients with schizophrenia. Expert Opin Drug Saf 2019; 18(12): 1149-60.
[http://dx.doi.org/10.1080/14740338.2019.1674809] [PMID: 31564170]

[60]   Delacrétaz A, Glatard A, Dubath C, *et al.* Psychotropic drug-induced genetic-epigenetic modulation of CRTC1 gene is associated with early weight gain in a prospective study of psychiatric patients. Clin Epigenetics 2019; 11(1): 198.
[http://dx.doi.org/10.1186/s13148-019-0792-0] [PMID: 31878957]

[61]   Di Lorenzo C, Pinto A, Ienca R, *et al.* A Randomized Double-Blind, Cross-Over Trial of very Low-Calorie Diet in Overweight Migraine Patients: A Possible Role for Ketones? Nutrients 2019; 11(8): 1742.
[http://dx.doi.org/10.3390/nu11081742] [PMID: 31357685]

[62]   Razeghi Jahromi S, Ghorbani Z, Martelletti P, Lampl C, Togha M. Association of diet and headache. J Headache Pain 2019; 20(1): 106.
[http://dx.doi.org/10.1186/s10194-019-1057-1] [PMID: 31726975]

[63]   Haynes A, Kersbergen I, Sutin A, Daly M, Robinson E. Does perceived overweight increase risk of depressive symptoms and suicidality beyond objective weight status? A systematic review and meta-analysis. Clin Psychol Rev 2019; 73101753
[http://dx.doi.org/10.1016/j.cpr.2019.101753] [PMID: 31715442]

[64]   Chao AM, Wadden TA, Berkowitz RI. Obesity in Adolescents with Psychiatric Disorders. Curr Psychiatry Rep 2019; 21(1): 3.
[http://dx.doi.org/10.1007/s11920-019-0990-7] [PMID: 30661128]

[65]   Gafoor R, Booth HP, Gulliford MC. Antidepressant utilisation and incidence of weight gain during 10 years' follow-up: population based cohort study. BMJ 2018; 361: k1951.
[http://dx.doi.org/10.1136/bmj.k1951] [PMID: 29793997]

[66]   Young WB, Rozen TD. Preventive treatment of migraine: effect on weight. Cephalalgia 2005; 25(1): 1-11.
[http://dx.doi.org/10.1111/j.1468-2982.2004.00819.x] [PMID: 15606563]

[67]   Hinze-Selch D, Schuld A, Kraus T, *et al.* Effects of antidepressants on weight and on the plasma levels of leptin, TNF-α and soluble TNF receptors: A longitudinal study in patients treated with amitriptyline or paroxetine. Neuropsychopharmacology 2000; 23(1): 13-9.
[http://dx.doi.org/10.1016/S0893-133X(00)00089-0] [PMID: 10869882]

[68]   Wang F, Wang J, Cao Y, Xu Z. Serotonin-norepinephrine reuptake inhibitors for the prevention of migraine and vestibular migraine: a systematic review and meta-analysis 2020.
[http://dx.doi.org/10.1136/rapm-2019-101207]

[69]   Young WB, Bradley KC, Anjum MW, Gebeline-Myers C. Duloxetine prophylaxis for episodic migraine in persons without depression: a prospective study. Headache 2013; 53(9): 1430-7.
[http://dx.doi.org/10.1111/head.12205] [PMID: 24032526]

[70]   Wofford MR, King DS, Harrell TK. Drug-induced metabolic syndrome. J Clin Hypertens (Greenwich) 2006; 8(2): 114-9.
[http://dx.doi.org/10.1111/j.1524-6175.2006.04751.x] [PMID: 16470080]

[71]   Akalestou E, Genser L, Rutter GA. Glucocorticoid Metabolism in Obesity and Following Weight Loss. Front Endocrinol (Lausanne) 2020; 11: 59.
[http://dx.doi.org/10.3389/fendo.2020.00059] [PMID: 32153504]

[72]   Bowles NP, Karatsoreos IN, Li X, *et al.* A peripheral endocannabinoid mechanism contributes to glucocorticoid-mediated metabolic syndrome. Proc Natl Acad Sci USA 2015; 112(1): 285-90.

[http://dx.doi.org/10.1073/pnas.1421420112] [PMID: 25535367]

[73] Armstrong MJ, Okun MS. Diagnosis and Treatment of Parkinson Disease: A Review. JAMA 2020; 323(6): 548-60.
[http://dx.doi.org/10.1001/jama.2019.22360] [PMID: 32044947]

[74] Martin-Jiménez CA, Gaitán-Vaca DM, Echeverria V, González J, Barreto GE. Relationship Between Obesity, Alzheimer's Disease, and Parkinson's Disease: an Astrocentric View. Mol Neurobiol 2017; 54(9): 7096-115.
[http://dx.doi.org/10.1007/s12035-016-0193-8] [PMID: 27796748]

[75] Sharma JC, Lewis A. Weight in Parkinson's Disease: Phenotypical Significance. Int Rev Neurobiol 2017; 134: 891-919.
[http://dx.doi.org/10.1016/bs.irn.2017.04.011] [PMID: 28805588]

[76] Bachmann CG, Zapf A, Brunner E, Trenkwalder C. Dopaminergic treatment is associated with decreased body weight in patients with Parkinson's disease and dyskinesias. Eur J Neurol 2009; 16(8): 895-901.
[http://dx.doi.org/10.1111/j.1468-1331.2009.02617.x] [PMID: 19374662]

[77] Gibson CD, Karmally W, McMahon DJ, Wardlaw SL, Korner J. Randomized pilot study of cabergoline, a dopamine receptor agonist: effects on body weight and glucose tolerance in obese adults. Diabetes Obes Metab 2012; 14(4): 335-40.
[http://dx.doi.org/10.1111/j.1463-1326.2011.01534.x] [PMID: 22074059]

[78] dos Santos Silva CM, Barbosa FR, Lima GA, *et al.* BMI and metabolic profile in patients with prolactinoma before and after treatment with dopamine agonists. Obesity (Silver Spring) 2011; 19(4): 800-5.
[http://dx.doi.org/10.1038/oby.2010.150] [PMID: 20559294]

[79] Graham KA, Gu H, Lieberman JA, Harp JB, Perkins DO. Double-blind, placebo-controlled investigation of amantadine for weight loss in subjects who gained weight with olanzapine. Am J Psychiatry 2005; 162(9): 1744-6.
[http://dx.doi.org/10.1176/appi.ajp.162.9.1744] [PMID: 16135638]

[80] Velazquez A, Apovian CM. Updates on obesity pharmacotherapy. Ann N Y Acad Sci 2018; 1411(1): 106-19.
[http://dx.doi.org/10.1111/nyas.13542] [PMID: 29377198]

[81] Saunders KH, Umashanker D, Igel LI, Kumar RB, Aronne LJ. Obesity Pharmacotherapy. Med Clin North Am 2018; 102(1): 135-48.
[http://dx.doi.org/10.1016/j.mcna.2017.08.010] [PMID: 29156182]

[82] Speyer H, Jakobsen AS, Westergaard C, *et al.* Lifestyle Interventions for Weight Management in People with Serious Mental Illness: A Systematic Review with Meta-Analysis, Trial Sequential Analysis, and Meta-Regression Analysis Exploring the Mediators and Moderators of Treatment Effects. Psychother Psychosom 2019; 88(6): 350-62.
[http://dx.doi.org/10.1159/000502293] [PMID: 31522170]

[83] Verhaegen AA, Van Gaal LF. Drugs That Affect Body Weight, Body Fat Distribution, and Metabolism.Endotext South Dartmouth (MA): MDTextcom, Inc. Feingold, KR 2019.

[84] Reynolds GP, McGowan OO. Mechanisms underlying metabolic disturbances associated with psychosis and antipsychotic drug treatment. J Psychopharmacol 2017; 31(11): 1430-6.
[http://dx.doi.org/10.1177/0269881117722987] [PMID: 28892404]

CHAPTER 3

Molecular Mechanism of Nervous System Disorders and Implications for New Therapeutic Targets

Farhin Patel and **Palash Mandal**[*]

Department of Biological Sciences, P. D. Patel Institute of Applied Sciences, Charotar University of Science and Technology, Changa, Anand- 388421, Gujarat, India

Abstract: The nervous system has a very good defence mechanism. The brain is protected by the skull, the spinal cord is shielded by vertebrae and thin membranes. The brain and spinal cord are buffered by cerebro-spinal fluid (CSF). The nervous system is susceptible to assorted disorders. It can be damaged by the structural defects, autoimmune disorders, infection, degeneration disorders, trauma, blood flow interference or tumors. At present, there is no treatment that can alleviate the disorders of the nervous system completely. In recent years, progress has been made in treating nervous system disorders symptomatically but still new product development is lagging behind in treating the disorders originating in the nervous system. This is due to several factors, including the intricacy of a particular disease or efficacy of the drug or delivering system to cross the blood-brain barrier (BBB). This chapter examines the modern state of major nervous system disorders like infection (meningitis), functional disorders (epilepsy, neuralgia), structural disorders (Bell's palsy, Guillain-Barre syndrome) and degeneration disorder (Huntington disease). The discussion topics include analysis of biological machinery underlying each disease, cytokine expression involved in each disease and how it is regulated in particular disease along with its involvement in targeted therapy, approved pharmaceutical drugs and the development of new therapeutic technologies or customized approaches for drug delivery to particular target (epigenetics, Gene therapy, stem cell therapy). We suppose that with the intensification of modern science, the mobility of nervous system disorders will decline.

Keywords: Bell's Palsy, Cytokines, Epigenetics, Guillain-Barre Syndrome, Huntington's Disease, Meningitis, Nervous system disorders, Neuralgia, Stem cell therapy.

---

[*] **Corresponding author Dr. Palash Mandal:** Department of Biological Sciences, P. D. Patel Institute of Applied Sciences, Charotar University of Science and Technology, Changa, Anand- 388421, Gujarat, India; Tel: +91-9666164654; Fax: 02697-247 100; E-mail: palashmandal.bio@charusat.ac.in

NERVOUS SYSTEM DISORDERS

The brain, spinal cord, and nerves make up the nervous system. Together, they control all the functions of the body [1].

(a) Brain and spinal cord: Central nervous system and

(b) Nerves in the rest of the body: Peripheral nervous system

The nervous system has a lot of protection. The brain is guarded by the skull, and spinal cord is shielded by vertebrae and membranes. They are cushioned by a clear fluid called cerebrospinal fluid (CSF) [1]. Damage to the nervous system, affects the communication between the brain, spinal cord and the body.

Infectious Disorders

Meningitis

Meningitis is a severe form of inflammation occurring in the membranes covering the spinal cord and brain, providing protection, such membrane is collectively called as the meninges [2].

Cause: The inflammation in the membranes may be caused by infection with bacteria, viruses, or any other organisms [3].

(a) Bacterial meningitis: Streptococcus pneumonia is a causative bacterium of meningitis [2].

(b) Virus meningitis: Viruses that cause meningitis include herpes simplex virus (type 2), enteroviruses, mumps virus, HIV (Human Immunodeficiency Virus) and varicella zoster virus [4]. Chronic recurrent form of herpes meningitis caused by herpes simplex virus type 2 is known as Mollaret's meningitis [5].

(c) Fungal meningitis: Cryptococcal meningitis is the most common fungal meningitis, which occurs due to *Cryptococcus neoformans* [6].

(d) Parasitic meningitis: Prevalence of eosinophils in the cerebrospinal fluid may cause parasitic meningitis [7].

Molecular Mechanism: The meninges comprise three membranes (Pia mater, arachnoid mater and dura mater) that, together with the CSF surrounds and protect the brain and spinal cord.

There are two routes to reach the meninges:

(A) Through direct contact between the meninges or blood stream

(B) Either by skin or nasal cavity

During inflammation, an organism that lives on the mucous surfaces (nasal cavity) disrupts the normal barrier and enters the bloodstream. Organism specifically enters the subarachnoid space in the membrane where the blood-brain barrier is defenseless (choroid plexus) [2]. Direct contamination of the CSF may arise from indwelling devices, skull fractures or infections of the nasopharynx/ nasal sinuses that made a tract with the subarachnoid space [2].

The big scale meninges inflammation during bacterial meningitis arises due to the entry of bacteria into the CNS in response to the immune system. When bacterial cell membrane components are identified by the astrocytes and microglia (brain immune cells), they release cytokines, hormone-like intermediaries that convert other brain immune cells and excite the other tissues to contribute in an immune response leading to more BBB (Blood Brain Barrier) permeability causing vasogenic cerebral edema. Interstitial edema occurs due to an increased number of WBCs (White blood cells) in the CSF leading to meninges inflammation. Cytotoxic edema occurs due to decreased blood flow in the CSF leading to inflamed blood vessel walls. Vasogenic cerebral edema, interstitial edema and cytotoxic edema, results in an increased intracranial pressure, leading to oxygen deprivation in the brain cells accounting programed cell death [2].

Diagnose: Diagnosing meningitis starts with health history and physical examination.

(a) Lumbar puncture (Spinal Tap): Sample of CSF is collected from the spinal canal through the insertion of needles. It can diagnose or exclude meningitis by observing an increased pressure in the central nervous system [8, 9].

(b) Blood Cultures: It helps in recognizing the bacteria in the blood and travel from the blood to the brain. Sepsis and meningitis are caused by *N. meningitidis* and *S. pneumonia.*

(c) Blood count: It verifies the count of red and white blood cells in the blood. White blood cells fight against infection. The complete blood count and C-reactive protein are usually higher in meningitis [9, 10].

(d) Chest X-ray: It will tell the presence of tuberculosis, fungal infections or pneumonia. Onset of meninges inflammation occurs after pneumonia.

(e) CT scans: Head CT scan may indicate the complications like brain inflammation or sinusitis. Bacteria can spread from the sinuses into the meninges [11].

Treatment: The first line of treatment in meninges inflammation is to treat with the antibiotics and antiviral drugs [8, 12]. Several other types of meningitis are preventable by having immunization with the Hib (Haemophilus influenzae type b), pneumococcal, mumps and meningococcal vaccines [2].

Epigenetics:

The modD gene (DNA methyltransferase) is responsible for phase switching of modD expression. modD- on/off variants have shown that modD regulates many expressions like infection, protection from the host and colonization. In modD-on variant, it also increased catalase enzyme expression conversing amplification in resistance to oxidative stress. The intonations of gene expression through the ModD phasevarion and its association with the hypervirulent clonal complex 41/44 (predominant cause of serogroup B meningococcal disease), provide a role in maintaining health and/or development of strains fitting to the clonal complex 41/44 [13].

Functional Disorders

Epilepsy

It is a central nervous system disorder showing the occurrence of epileptic seizure due to abnormal brain activity [14].

Cause: The epilepsy disorder does not contain any perceptible cause, but it is divided into two factors:

a. Genetic factors: The genes involved in the epileptic seizures are GABA (Gamma-aminobutyric acid), GPCR (G protein-coupled receptor), ion channels receptors and enzymes [15].
b. Acquired factors: Epilepsy may occur due to other conditions like head trauma, brain tumors or stroke, infectious diseases like meningitis, AIDS (Acquired ImmunoDeficiency Syndrome), prenatal injury or developmental disorders like autism [16, 17].

Molecular Mechanism: The exact mechanism behind epilepsy is unknown [18]. Only a few steps are known, *i.e.* its cellular and network mechanisms [18].

a. First mechanism: The change in ion channel receptors or ion concentrations or dysfunction of inhibitory neurons results in the resistance of excitatory neurons during that period. This leads to seizures in specific areas called as "seizure focus" [19].

b. Second mechanism: Occurrence of secondary epileptic conditions occurs through the process called as epileptogenesis in which there is a down-regulation of inhibitory circuits or up-regulation of excitatory circuits following the brain injury [20, 21].

c. Third mechanism: BBB dysfunction will allow the substances in blood to enter the brain [22].

Diagnosis: It is typically based on the onset of seizures and its cause behind it [23].

a. Electroencephalogram (EEG): Observe the abnormal patterns of brain waves.

b. CT scan or MRI: It will observe the structure of the brain.

Cytokines Involved in Epilepsy:

S100ß (astrocyte- derived cytokine): It stimulates neurite growth. Serotonin 5-HT receptors expressed by astrocytes binds with serotonin (neurotransmitter) and helps in releasing S100ß and further encourage the progression of serotonergic neuritis. There is an increase in astrrocytic intracellular calcium levels, which may indirectly affect calcium levels of neurons [24].

IL-6: Patients with temporal lobe epilepsy showed increased IL-6 (Interleukin-6) levels after seizure and levels remain elevated for 24 hrs [25].

IL-1β: Case study showed that epileptic patients taking valproate had higher levels of IL-1β (Interleukin- 1 beta) compared to patients not treated with Valproate (VPA) [26].

IL-1: *In- vivo* study model, Interleukin-1 (IL-1) prolongs the duration of kainic acid-induced EEG seizures. IL-1 Converting Enzyme (ICE) inhibitors inhibit the IL-1 production and delays epilepsy onset along with a reduction in seizure number and duration. At the location of hippocampal pyramidal neurons, IL-1R1 colocalizes with NMDA receptors and facilitates tyrosine phosphorylation of IL-1β of the NR2B subunit by activating Src kinases. As a result, there is an up-regulation of NMDA receptor- mediated Ca^{2+} influx stimulating excitotoxicity into neurons and probably in the generation of seizure [27].

Treatment: The following are the treatments available for epilepsy (Table **1**).

Table 1. Treatment availability for epilepsy.

Treatment	Medication	References
Anticonvulsant	Phenobarbital, Phenytoin, Carbamazepine and VPA.	[28]
Surgery	Sectioning of hippocampus through anterior temporal lobe resection, tumor removal and sectioning of neocortex part. Corpus Callosotomy: It is done to decrease the number of seizures.	[29]
Stimulation of neurons	Anterior thalamic stimulation, Closed- loop responsive stimulation and vagus nerve stimulation	[30, 31]

Gene Therapy: With the aim of targeting DNA or RNA to the epileptogenic area, the practice of viral vector gene transfer seems to be promising. Transgenes used for the treatment of epilepsy are neuropeptides (somatostatin, galanin, and neuropeptide Y), ion channels (potassium channels) and neurotransmitter receptors (adenosine and gamma-aminobutryic acid (GABA) receptors) [32 - 36] (Fig. **1**). Among vectors are adenovirus and adeno-associated virus vectors (AAV) and even lentiviral vectors are used in gene therapy [37].

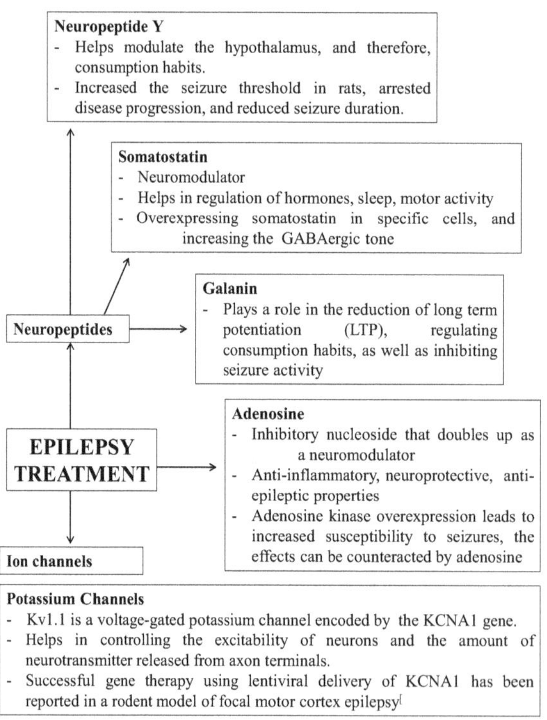

Fig. (1). Gene therapy for epileptic seizures.

• Seizure-suppressant strategies are as follows:

1. Silencing of endogenous excitatory cells, or

2. Activating endogenous GABAergic interneurons.

In epileptic foci of the brain, both seizure- suppressant strategies may regulate hyperexcitability. Currently, probable entrants for the neuronal silencing approach include alternate of the light-driven ion pump, Halorhodopsin (NpHR), and light-driven proton pumps, such as Archaerhodopsin (Arch) and Bacteriorhodopsin (BR). The study demonstrated that illumination of yellow light on the NpHR-transduced neurons in organotypic slice culture, could efficiently and repetitively block epileptiform activity induced by electrical stimulation. This data suggested that in chronic epileptic *in-vivo* model, NpHR activation can suppress or block seizures. In GABAergic interneurons, expression of channelrhodopsin (ChR2) would allow for their light activation. This resulted in an up-regulated GABAergic transmission onto major neurons to which GABAergic interneurons are connected synaptically which inhibit major neurons [38].

Neuralgia

It is a disease caused by irritated or damaged nerves due to stabbing, sweltering or severe pain [39]. There are three types of neuralgia *i.e.* trigeminal neuralgia, glossopharyngeal neuralgia and intercostal neuralgia [39].

Types of Neuralgia

1. Trigminal neuralgia: It is connected with pain from the trigeminal nerve, which travels from the brain and spreads to various parts of the face. It can also be caused by multiple sclerosis, injury to the nerve, or other causes [40].

2. Glossopharyngeal neuralgia: It is related to the pain of glossopharyngeal nerve present in the throat. It also produces pain in the neck [40].

3. Intercostal neuralgia: It occurs due to the onset of shingles leading to painful rashes and blisters anywhere on the body. It will always occur along the path of a nerve, so it is usually isolated to one side of the body [40].

Cause: The proper cause of nerve pain is poorly understood. Some of the common causes are as follows (Table **2**).

Table 2. The common causes of the neuropathic pain.

	Type of Neuralgia	Cause	Reference
Infection	Postherpetic neuralgia (PHN)	• Shingles – caused by chicken pox	[41]
Pressure on a nerve	Trigeminal neuralgia	• Multiple sclerosis is caused by deterioration of myelin covering the nerves. • Pressure of a swollen blood vessel	[41]
Nerve damage	Neuralgia	• Diabetes- the excess glucose in the bloodstream may damage nerves	[41]

Molecular Mechanism: By considering the neuroplastic modifications along with neuron damage, scientists may be able to improve the hyperexcitability mechanism in the entire nervous system which is said to cause neuropathic pain [42].

(A). Peripheral Nerve Injury

Severity of the brain injury can lead to the determination of traumatic response to neurons. This response can be categorized by Seddon's classification. In this classification, nerve injury is described as neurotmesis, axonotmesis or neurapraxia. Following traumatic injury to the nerve, there is injury discharge occurring, *i.e.* initiation of afferent impulses. This directly linked to the inception of neuropathic pain [43] (Fig. **2**).

(B). Central Nerve Injury

Neuronal injury in the CNS leads to local degeneration of the axonal nerve and the myelin sheath (Fig. **3**).

Cytokines Involved in Neuralgia: Patients with PHN Postherpetic neuralgia (PHN), serum $CD3^+$ (pan-T lymphocytes), $CD4^+$ (helper/inducer), and $CD8^+$ (suppressor/cytotoxic) lymphocytes was reduced considerably when compared with normal control. Patients with acute phase herpes zoster (HZ) and has developed PHN showed a significant elevation in the levels of IL-1β, IL-6, TNF-α (Tumor necrosis factor- alpha), IL-8, and IL-10 compared to control. IL-6 was significantly higher in the patients with acute phase herpes zoster and developed PHN compared with patients having only acute phase HZ and not developed PHN [44].

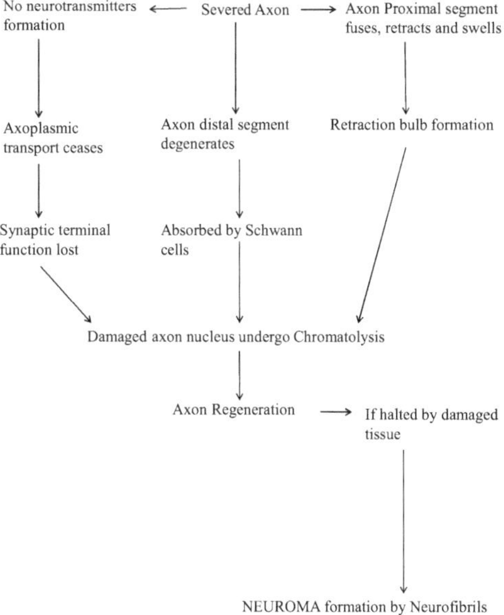

Fig. (2). Biological mechanism behind the peripheral nerve injury.

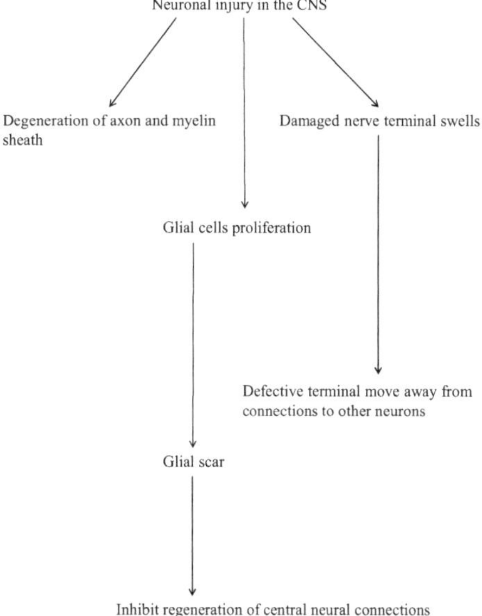

Fig. (3). Biological mechanism behind the central nerve injury.

Diagnosis: Diagnosis involved following tests:

(a) Electromyography (EMG) test or nerve conduction test: Recognizing the missing sensory or motor neurons to identify damaged nerves.

Nerve conduction test: Peripheral nerve is stimulated through a technique called microneurography.The results are recorded from the purely sensory area of the nerve [45, 46].

(b) McGill Pain Questionnaire: This will assess neuralgia through physical and experimental examination, history and description of pain [47].

• Physical examination includes test response to stimuli like touch, vibration and temperature.

(c) Type of stimuli: Mechanical, chemical or thermal responses is elicited depending on the type of stimuli [43].

(d) Laser evoked potentials: Using lasers, it will stimulate the thermonociceptors in the skin to measure the cortical responses [48].

(e) Punch skin biopsy: It will quantify A- delta nerve fibers and nerve fiber C. It will measure the density of intra-epidermal nerve fibers to quantify [46].

Treatment: Specific medications are available to treat the neuralgia:

(a) Antidepressant medication: Cymbalta

(b) Antiepileptic medication: Lyrica

(c) Anticonvulsant medications: It is used to block nerve shooting [45, 49].

(d) Gabapentin: This drug proved to be efficacious in the treatment of postherpetic neuralgia [50].

(e) Resveratrol: It is an effectual 5' adenosine monophosphate-activated protein kinase (AMPK) activators used for the treatment of chronic trigeminal neuralgia. It helps by preventing glia activation and release glia-mediated neuroinflammation [51].

Resveratrol activates AMPK in the spinal glia, resulted in the treatment of tumor cell implantation-induced neuroinflammation. Resveratrol inhibits chronic constriction injury (CCI)- evoked activation of astrocyte and microglial and upturned the production of IL-1β and TNF-α *via* the activation of AMPK [51].

Oral administration of resveratrol downregulated the mitogen-activated protein kinase (MAPK or MAP kinase) expression levels. Therefore, resveratrol suppresses the MAPK activation signalling pathway by inhibiting the microglial activation providing anti- neuroinflammatory effect [51].

(f) Vitamin C: Constituent used as a substitute therapeutic strategy in the HZ treatment [52].

Gene Therapy:

Trigeminal pain

In a mouse model with inflammatory pain, administration of the enkephalin-expressing vector gives protection to the respective model, but does not result in complete loss in normal perception [53].

Epigenetics:

HDAC (Histone Deacetylase) inhibitors and HAT (Histone Acetyltransferase) inhibitors are the most commonly used epigenetic drugs in neuropathic pain studies (Table **3**).

Table 3. HDAC and HAT inhibitors as epigenetic modulators in neuropathic pain.

HDAC Inhibitors	Role	Reference
Valproic acid (VPA) and Trichostatin A (TSA)	It prevents partial sciatic nerve ligation (PSNL) –induced hypoesthesia	[54]
MS-275	It prevents Spinal Nerve Ligation (SNL)-induced mechanical and thermal hyperalgesia by increasing acetylation of H3K9 and altering HDAC1 expression in the dorsal horn of the spinal cord	[55]
HAT Inhibitors	**Role**	**Reference**
Anacardic acid	Decreased acetylation of H3K9 at the promoters of macrophage inflammatory protein 2 and CXC chemokine receptor type 2 in macrophages and neutrophils infiltrating the injured tissue, thereby attenuating Partial sciatic nerve ligation (PSNL)-induced thermal hyperalgesia	[56]
p300 short hairpin RNA or C646	Reversed CCI (chronic constriction injury) - induced mechanical allodynia and thermal hyperalgesia	[57]
Curcumin	Silence pronociceptive genes *Bdnf* and cyclooxygenase (COX) -2 by reducing the binding of p300/cAMP response element-binding protein (CREB)-binding protein, H3K9ac, and H4K5ac to their promoters and attenuates neuropathic pain	[58]

Structural Disorder

Bell's Palsy (Idiopathic Facial Paralysis)

It is a type of facial palsy, which can occur at any stage. It is a facial paralysis which results in an incapability to control the facial muscles on that particular side [59].

Cause: The exact reason behind Ball palsy is still unknown. But it is correlated with viral infection. Some viruses which are linked to it are as follows [60] (Table 4).

Table 4. Various viruses linked to Bell's palsy.

Types of Viruses	Diseases
Herpes zoster (HZ)	Chickenpox and shingles
Herpes simplex	Cold sores and genital herpes
Epstein-Barr	Infectious mononucleosis
Cytomegalovirus	Cytomegalovirus infections
Influenza B	Flu
Rubella	German measles
Adenovirus	Respiratory illnesses
Mumps virus	Mumps
Coxsackievirus	Hand-foot-and-mouth disease

Molecular Mechanism: This disorder occurs due to a facial nerve fault, *i.e.* VII cranial nerve, whose role is to control the facial muscles. Facial nerve become swollen and inflamed- usually related to infection caused by specific viruses as mentioned above. The inflamed facial nerve builds a pressure on the nerve where it exits the skull within the stylomastoid foramen leading to a blocking the transmission of neuronal signalling or may damage the nerve. The facial paralysis belongs to the infranuclear or lower motor neuron type. The herpes simplex virus type 1 (HSV-1) infection is associated with demyelination of nerves [61].

In-vivo model of facial palsy, Aquaporin-1 (AQP-1) protein levels were increased drastically after inoculation of HSV-1 [38]. *In-vitro* hypoxia model of Schwann cells, U0126 (extracellular signal-regulated kinase (ERK) antagonist) inhibit the up-regulation of phosphorylated ERK and AQP-1 along with morphological modifications of Schwann cells. Therefore, in the Bell palsy mouse model, it was assumed that the combined effect of up-regulation of phosphorylated ERK with facial palsy induced by HSV-1, there might be ERK- MAPK pathway involved in the elevated levels of AQP-1 [62].

Cytokines Involved in Bell's Palsy: In Bell's palsy, up-regulated levels of cytokines like IL-6, IL-8, and TNF-α signifies as a pathogenic factor [63].

Decreased levels of total T cells, CD3 and CD4 (T helper/inducing cells) have been found in the acute phase of Bell's palsy. Within 24 days from the clinical onset of Bell's palsy, there is a decreased level of peripheral blood T lymphocyte and an elevated levels of B lymphocyte [62].

Diagnosis: There are no specific tests or scanning required for making the diagnosis. The degree of damage to the nerve can be measured using the House-Brackmann score [64].

Infection with the herpes zoster virus involves the facial nerve damage. This infection is difficult to eliminate through differential diagnosis. Recurrence of current herpes zoster infection leads to facial paralysis in a Bell's palsy type pattern is recognized as Ramsay Hunt syndrome type 2. The Bell's palsy's may be produce by Lyme disease (it is caused by the bacteria named *Borrelia burgdorferi* and is transmitted to humans through the bite of infected blacklegged ticks or deer ticks) [65].

Treatment: The following are few known managements used to treat Bell's palsy (Table **5**).

Table 5. Drugs used in the treatment of Bell's palsy.

Treatment	Drug	Reference
Steroids	Prednisone (corticosteroids)	[64, 66]
Antivirals	Aciclovir	[67]
Physiotherapy	To stimulate the facial nerve and to maintain muscle tendency of the particular damaged facial muscles	[68]
Surgerical facial nerve decompression	Surgical decompression medial to the geniculate ganglion significantly improves the chances of normal or near-normal return of facial function	[69]

Guillain–Barré Syndrome (GBS)

It is a rare disorder caused by the peripheral nervous system damaged due to the immune system attack. The preliminary symptoms are muscle weakness and tingling sensation in the extremities and eventually it spreads and paralyzes the entire body [70].

Cause: The exact cause of GBS is unknown. This particular disorder appears after the onset of following symptoms like respiratory tract or stomach flu (gastroenteritis) infection. Newly, there have been a few reports following the subsequent infection with the Zika virus [71, 72]. Other than Zika virus, herpes viruses like HHV- 4 and HHV-3 have been associated with GBS. Nearly, one-fourth cases of GBS are triggered by *Campylobacter jejuni* bacteria and few with *Mycoplasma pneumonia.* Few reports are marked by the presence of cytomegalovirus (CMV, HHV-5) [73] (Fig. **4**).

Molecular Mechanism: Immune system attacks the nerves resulting into the demyelination of myelin sheath by WBCs (T lymphocytes and macrophages). Further leads to the activation of a complement system (blood proteins). In contrast, the axonal variant is facilitated by IgG antibodies and complement against the cell membrane covering the axon with indirect involvement of lymphocyte [73]. Various antibodies bind to gangliosides (GM1, GD1a, GT1a and GQ1b). After the infection, the production of particular antibodies has been associated with the immune system reacting with microbial bodies as well as it will as also reacts with materials present naturally in the body [73, 74]. After a *Campylobacter* infection, the body produces antibodies of the IgA class; only a small proportion of people also produce IgG antibodies against bacterial cell wall substances (*e.g.* lipooligosaccharides) that cross react with human nerve cell gangliosides [74].

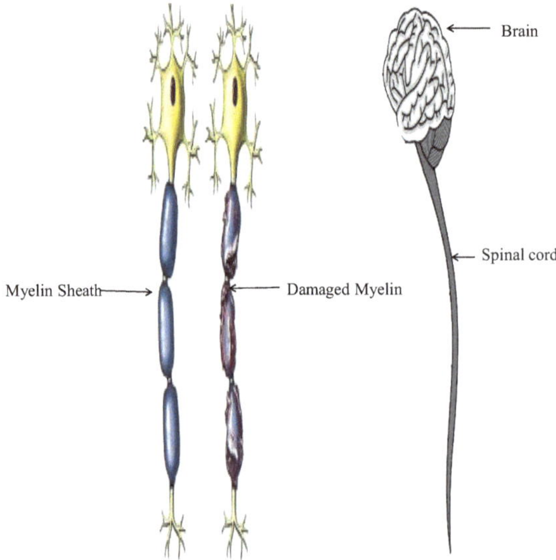

Fig. (4). The cause behind Guillain–Barré syndrome.

Cytokines Involved in GBS: The following cytokines play a potential role in GBS pathogenesis (Table **6**).

Table 6. Cytokines involved in GBS.

Interferon gamma (IFN-γ)	In GBS patients, serum IFN-γ levels was elevated. Peripheral blood mononuclear cells (PBMC), secreting IFN-γ levels were elevated in 25% of GBS patients, which specified immunopathological role of T cells in GBS. In GBS patients, auto- antibodies neutralization to IFN-γ were associated with down-regulation of IFN-γ producing cells and with better clinical disability. In GBS, IFN-γ has ability to convert peripheral CD4(+)CD25(-) T cells to CD4(+)CD25(+) regulatory T cells.	[75 - 77]
TNF- α	In GBS patients, serum TNF- α was elevated. TNF- α converting enzyme (TACE) levels were elevated, In GBS patients, processing of membrane-bound inactive pro- TNF- α into the active soluble cytokine TNF- α. Following Intravenous Immunoglobulin (IVIg) treatment, sTNFR1 expression was increased while TNF-α and TNF- α receptor 1 (TNFR1, p55) expression levels were decreased. TNF- α and (TNFR2, p75) TNFR2 expression levels were elevated after IVIg treatment. TNF- α –TNFR2 stimulates expansion and function of mouse CD49(+)CD25(+) Tregs cells.	[78 - 81]
Interleukin- 12	In the serum of AIDP (acute inflammatory demyelinating polyradiculoneuropathy) patient, elevated levels of IL-12 and IL-12R on PBMCs were found and decreased levels of IL-12R were seen after the IVIg treatment. In GBS patients, IL-23p19 protein was measured in CSF.	[76, 82]
IL-1β	In GBS patients, IL-1β was identified in CSF. In sural nerve biopsies, elevated expression levels of IL-1β were immunolocalized on Schwann cells (SC) membranes.	[83, 84]
Interleukin- 18	In GBS patients, IL-18 act as co-inducer of Th1 and Th2 cytokine. Serum IL-18 was increased in GBS patients.	[85]
IL-6	In GBs patients, serum and CSF levels of IL-6 were up-regulated.	[86, 87]
Transforming growth factor-β (TGF-β)	During the recovery of GBS, decreased levels of decreased expression levels of TGF-β1 cytokine were observed and TGF- β1 mRNA expression level was found to be increased. Significant elevated levels of TGF-β secreting cells were observed in the acute phase of GBS.	[88]
Interleukin- 10	In the acute phase of GBS, IL10-secreting bone marrow nucleated cells (BMNC) expression levels were elevated. IL-10 worsens the disease *via* enhancing the ganglioside Antibody (Ab) production probably.	[89, 90]

(Table 6) cont.....

| Interleukin- 4 | During acute and recovery phase of GBS, serum levels of IL-4 were increased. | [91] |
| Chemokines Monocyte chemoattractant protein (MCP)-1 and Gamma-interferon inducible protein IP-10 | Increased CSF levels of MCP-1 and IL-10 were observed prior to IVIg treatment in GBS Patients with acute phase. | [92] |

Diagnosis: The diagnosis of GBS depends on outcomes such as muscle weakness or paralysis, no fever, absence of reflexes and a other symptoms

1. Cerebrospinal fluid analysis (through a lumbar spinal puncture)

2. Nerve conduction studies [93, 94]

3. Blood tests: Potassium and sodium

(a) Blood potassium level: Lower levels; to exclude the other possibility of muscle weakness.

(b) Blood sodium level: Low level in the blood is often related with GBS. This leads to unsuitable secretion of antidiuretic hormone (ADH) resulting in the retention of water [95].

4. MRI: In the spinal cord, MRI is performed to distinguish the symptoms like limb weakness caused due to GBS or other illness [93]. If results showed an enhancement of nerve roots, then it's a sign of GBS [93].

Treatment: The following are the respective treatment of GBS (Table **7**).

Table 7. Respective treatment of Guillain–Barré syndrome.

Treatment	Function	Reference
Immunotherapy	(a) Plasmapheresis: It will reduce the immune system attack on the nerves by filtering antibodies out of the blood. (b) Intravenous immunoglobulins (IVIG): It will neutralize the dangerous antibodies and inflammation.	[96]
Ventilation	In case of respiratory failure, intubation of the trachea is also required and worst case mechanical ventilation is needed. Ventilator support can be predicted by measurement of two spirometry-based breathing tests: the forced vital capacity (FVC) and the negative inspiratory force (NIF).	[97]

(Table 7) cont.....

NOVEL POSSIBLE APPROACHES		
Stem cell therapy	10 year old girl diagnosed with chronic GBS. Before the treatment: She was not able to walk for a few meters without falling down or move her hands. Therapy: Four Umbilical Cord Blood Stem Cell Injections After the treatment: She was able to walk almost 2000 meters without falling down. Her hand mobility got even better.	[98]
Targeting CD11b or alpha M integrin	At the beginning of GBS, blocking or inhibiting CD11b can limit or reduce the amount of abnormal leukocyte trafficking, inflammation. This results in demyelination and loss of axons in Acute inflammatory demyelinating polyneuropathy (AIDP) patients From blood circulation, selectively removing CD11b leukocytes, so that CD11b leukocytes are not available for adhering to the blood-nerve barrier endothelial cells in patient's nerves to treat GBS.	[99]
Modulation of cytokine pathway	IL-12 activated Th1 cells *via* the Janus kinase (JAK) 2/Signal transducer and activator of transcription protein (STAT) 4 pathway IL-4 activated Th2 cells *via* JAK1-3/STAT6. Targeting Nuclear factor kappa-light-chain-enhancer of activated B cells (NF-κB) can be potential molecular therapy in autoimmune disease. Suppression of Interleukin- 23 and IL-1-driven Interleukin- 17 production by inhibiting ERK- MAPK signaling pathway and attenuates autoimmune disease. AKT axis signaling can be smart therapeutic strategy in targeting autoimmune disease.	[100 - 105]
Blockage of cytokines by monoclonal antibodies (mAb) and fusion proteins	Anti-TNF-α mAb and sTNFR, IL-1bR antagonist, anti-IL-6RmAb are effective in the treatment of autoimmune disease. Blocking IL- 12/IL- 23 by inducing drugs like ABT-84, Apilimod, CNTO-1275 are clinically tested in GBS. Blocking IFN- γ can be a potential target for GBS.	[106 - 110]
Cytokines for neuroprotection and regeneration	IFN-γ, TNF-α, IL-6 induce auto-reactive T cell apoptosis IFN-γ, TGF-β, IL-10 retain Treg cell levels; IL-1, IL-6, IFN-γ induce Schwann cells (SC) proliferation; IL-10 reduces the neuropathic pain and enhance nerve repair. Increased GM- 1 ganglioside specific T cell reactivity and its related cytokine might have an immuno-regulatory or neuro-protective effect.	[111]

Degenerative Disorder

Neurodegeneration is the advanced loss of structural or functional neurons, including loss of neurons.

Huntington's Disease

Huntington's disease (HD) is a lethal genetic neurodegenerative disease that causes the progressive failure of neurons in the brain [112]. It is also called as the archetypal family disease because it is inherited from an individual's parents [113].

Cause: HD is a genetic disease caused by mutation in the Huntingtin gene (HTT) [112]., It's an important gene, which is needed to produce a protein called huntingtin [113]. This protein is needed by the neurons for the development of body before birth [113]. It is caused by polyglutamine expansion in the first exon of the HTT gene.

A mutation in the huntingtin gene involves a DNA segment containing a CAG (cytosine-adenine-guanine) trinucleotide repeat [92]. In a normal person, CAG segment is repeated 10 to 35 times within the gene, while it is repeated more than 40 times in HD people [114].

Molecular Mechanism: Mutant HTT gives rise to an elongated polyglutamine tract at the amino terminus of the translated HTT protein [115]. These fragments of protein undergo aggregation and misfolding leading to fibrillary aggregates [116]. These aggregates accumulate to form inclusion bodies within cells, resulting in neuronal dysfunction [116, 117].

Mutant HTT protein leads to mitochondrial dysfunction [118]. The impairment of electron transport chain in the mitochondria leads to an increased levels of oxidative stress. Therefore, there is a release of reactive oxygen species (ROS) [119].

Altered HTT protein along with other proteins in neurons results in an increased susceptibility of neurotransmitter called glutamine. Glutamine, even in normal amount, can cause excitotoxins to be expressed because of increased susceptibility [116] (Fig. **5**).

Therapeutic Approaches:

(A). Mitochondria-directed Therapies

Treatment of creatine reduces the serum level of 8-hydroxy-2′deoxyguanosine (indicates oxidative damage to DNA) [120]. It is being reported that injection of (R)-alpha-lipoic acid (LA) significantly improved glutathione redox status in both myocardial and cerebral tissues of old rats when compared to normal rats [121]. A study on ApoE4 mice showed suggestively improved cognitive function when administered with LA and ALCAR (acetyl-L-carnitine- transporter of acetyl groups across the mitochondrial membrane) [122].

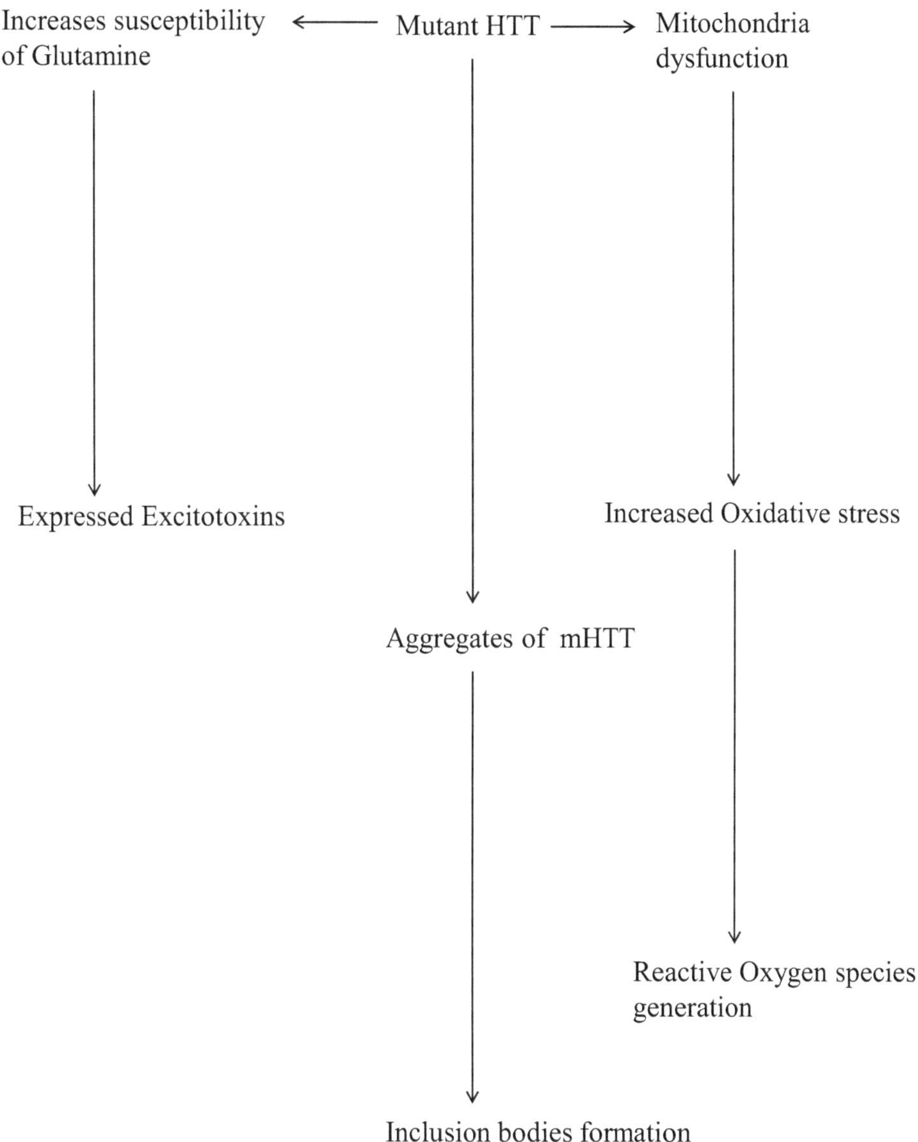

Fig. (5). Biological mechanism of Huntington disease.

(B). Stem Cell Therapy

Cell based therapy: In animals, injection of kainic acid (analogs of glutamic acid) was given to develop HD model showing lesioned striatum development. The transplantation of fetal rat striatal tissue fragments showed improved behavioral activity. The embryonic striatal tissues have been transplanted in excitotoxic striatal lesioned HD model and showed graft survival and expressed normal straiatum cellular markers of different ranges [123 - 126]. Possible approach of this therapy was to block neuronal dysfunction or to replace lost neurons in the striatum [127].

On HD patient, a pilot study was conducted by transplantating fetal stratium. The result revealed improved cognitive functions and graft survival within the striatum without displacing the surrounding tissue [128, 129].

(C). Neural Stem Cell Therapy

Mutant HTT leads to GABAergic neuron death in striatum [130, 131]. *In-vivo*, QA (quinolinic acid: analog of glutamic acid) - HD model, researchers transplanted GABAergic neurons isolated from neural stem/progenitor cell (NSC) line, using retinoic acid and KCl (potassium chloride) depolarization resulting in an improved functional deficits and cell survival [125].

Transplantation of F3 human NSCs secretes brain- derived neurotrophic factor (BDNF) results in behavioral and anatomical recovery in HD models [132]. NSCs intensified the production of nerve growth factor (NGF) leading to neuron protection in HD patients [133]. Transplantation of NSC leads to striatal atrophy reduction, improved functional recovery and prevent tissue loss [134].

In QA-HD model, transplantation of bone marrow mesenchymal stem cell showed improved behavioral function. The grafted cells release some growth factors which allowed the survival of host cells and facilitate the other compensatory responses [135].

Migration of NSCs in HD pathological lesions followed systematic administrative mechanism. It was shown that transplanted NSCs are conscripted by selective chemoattractant signals produced at central nervous system (CNS) sites, such as vascular endothelial cell growth factor (VEGF), stem cell factor (SCF) and stromal cell derived factor- 1 (SDF- 1) [136 - 138].

(D). Epigenetic Modulators

In *Drosophila* HD models, researchers identified the HDACi by alleviating neurodegeneration [139]. In HD patients, H2AFY (histone variant macroH2A1) protein levels was reduced when treated with HDACi [140]. In R6/2 HD transgenic mice model, researchers target Histone methylation by administering Nogalamycin, which showed decreased H3K9me3 levels with the chromatin remodelling resulting in slow disease progression [141].

(E). Mitochondrial Dynamics Modulators

P110, an inhibitory peptide blocking Dynamin-related protein 1 (Drp1) and Mitochondrial fission 1 (Fis 1) interaction, attenuates HD-associated neurotoxicity and behaviour deficits [142].

CONCLUSION

The nervous system is a multifaceted, extremely specific network. It systematizes, enlightens, and guides the interactions among the human frame. The recent developments in the fields of nervous system disorders are grounded on directing the degenerative progressions that lead to the neuronal death. Because of the complexity involved in respective nervous system disorders, scientists have recognized a few potential treatments. At present, many beneficial therapeutic approaches have been proposed to treat/ prevent the signs of nervous system disorders. Yet there subsists a gap for the active therapies for curing the nervous system disorders. Hence, few therapeutic approaches like epigenetics, gene therapy, stem cell therapy, mitochondrial regulators may provide the evidence in treating the respective nervous system disorders.

CONSENT FOR PUBLICATION

Not applicable.

CONFLICT OF INTEREST

The author confirms that this chapter content has no conflict of interest.

ACKNOWLEDGEMENTS

Declared none.

REFERENCES

[1]   Nervous System Diseases | Neurologic Diseases | MedlinePlus. Retrieved 2018-02-02 2003.

[2]   Sáez-Llorens X, McCracken GH Jr. Bacterial meningitis in children. Lancet 2003; 361(9375): 2139-48.
        [http://dx.doi.org/10.1016/S0140-6736(03)13693-8] [PMID: 12826449]

[3]   Ginsberg L. Difficult and recurrent meningitis. J Neurol Neurosurg Psychiatry 2004; 75 (Suppl. 1): i16-21.
        [http://dx.doi.org/10.1136/jnnp.2003.034272] [PMID: 14978146]

[4]   Logan SA, MacMahon E. Viral meningitis. BMJ 2008; 336(7634): 36-40.
        [http://dx.doi.org/10.1136/bmj.39409.673657.AE] [PMID: 18174598]

[5]   Shalabi M, Whitley RJ. Recurrent benign lymphocytic meningitis. Clin Infect Dis 2006; 43(9): 1194-7.
        [http://dx.doi.org/10.1086/508281] [PMID: 17029141]

[6]   Kauffman CA, Pappas PG, Sobel JD, Dismukes WE. Essentials of clinical mycology. 2nd ed; p. 77.. New York: Springer 2011 2016.

[7]   Graeff-Teixeira C, da Silva AC, Yoshimura K. Update on eosinophilic meningoencephalitis and its clinical relevance. Clin Microbiol Rev 2009; 22(2): 322-48.
        [http://dx.doi.org/10.1128/CMR.00044-08] [PMID: 19366917]

[8]   "Bacterial Meningitis" CDC 1 April 2014 Archived from the original on 5 March 2016 Retrieved 5 March 2016.

[9]   Tunkel AR, Hartman BJ, Kaplan SL, *et al.* Practice guidelines for the management of bacterial meningitis. Clin Infect Dis 2004; 39(9): 1267-84.
        [http://dx.doi.org/10.1086/425368] [PMID: 15494903]

[10]   Chaudhuri A, Martinez-Martin P, Kennedy PG, *et al.* EFNS guideline on the management of community-acquired bacterial meningitis: report of an EFNS Task Force on acute bacterial meningitis in older children and adults. Eur J Neurol 2008; 15(7): 649-59.
        [http://dx.doi.org/10.1111/j.1468-1331.2008.02193.x] [PMID: 18582342]

[11]   Hasbun R, Abrahams J, Jekel J, Quagliarello VJ. Computed tomography of the head before lumbar puncture in adults with suspected meningitis. N Engl J Med 2001; 345(24): 1727-33.
        [http://dx.doi.org/10.1056/NEJMoa010399] [PMID: 11742046]

[12]   Viral Meningitis" CDC 26 November 2014 Archived from the original on 4 March 2016 Retrieved 5 March 2016.

[13]   Seib KL, Pigozzi E, Muzzi A, *et al.* A novel epigenetic regulator associated with the hypervirulent Neisseria meningitidis clonal complex 41/44. FASEB J 2011; 25(10): 3622-33.
        [http://dx.doi.org/10.1096/fj.11-183590] [PMID: 21680891]

[14]   Fisher RS, van Emde Boas W, Blume W, *et al.* Epileptic seizures and epilepsy: definitions proposed by the International League Against Epilepsy (ILAE) and the International Bureau for Epilepsy (IBE). Epilepsia 2005; 46(4): 470-2.
        [http://dx.doi.org/10.1111/j.0013-9580.2005.66104.x] [PMID: 15816939]

[15]   Greenberg DA, Aminoff MJ, Simon RP. Movement Disorders.Clinical Neurology, 8e. New York: McGraw-Hill 2012.

[16]   Niedermeyer E. The epilepsies: diagnosis and management. Baltimore: Urban & Schwarzenberg 1990.

[17]   World Health Organization (WHO). Epilepsy: epidemiology, aetiology and prognosis. 2012.

[18]   Jasper HH. Jasper's basic mechanisms of the epilepsies. OUP USA; 2012 Jun 29.

[19]   McPhee SJ, Ganong WF. Pathophysiology of Disease: An Introduction to Clinical Medicine, diterjemahkan oleh Brahm U. Jakarta: EGC 2010; pp. 493-500.

[20]   Goldberg EM, Coulter DA. Mechanisms of epileptogenesis: a convergence on neural circuit dysfunction. Nat Rev Neurosci 2013; 14(5): 337-49.
        [http://dx.doi.org/10.1038/nrn3482] [PMID: 23595016]

[21]   Oby E, Janigro D. The blood-brain barrier and epilepsy. Epilepsia 2006; 47(11): 1761-74.
        [http://dx.doi.org/10.1111/j.1528-1167.2006.00817.x] [PMID: 17116015]

[22]   Kwan P, Brodie MJ. Definition of refractory epilepsy: defining the indefinable? Lancet Neurol 2010; 9(1): 27-9.
        [http://dx.doi.org/10.1016/S1474-4422(09)70304-7] [PMID: 19914135]

[23]   Newton CR, Garcia HH. Epilepsy in poor regions of the world. Lancet 2012; 380(9848): 1193-201.
[http://dx.doi.org/10.1016/S0140-6736(12)61381-6] [PMID: 23021288]

[24]   Griffin WS, Yeralan O, Sheng JG, *et al.* Overexpression of the neurotrophic cytokine S100 β in human temporal lobe epilepsy. J Neurochem 1995; 65(1): 228-33.
[http://dx.doi.org/10.1046/j.1471-4159.1995.65010228.x] [PMID: 7790864]

[25]   Liimatainen S, Fallah M, Kharazmi E, Peltola M, Peltola J. Interleukin-6 levels are increased in temporal lobe epilepsy but not in extra-temporal lobe epilepsy. J Neurol 2009; 256(5): 796-802.
[http://dx.doi.org/10.1007/s00415-009-5021-x] [PMID: 19252806]

[26]   Bauer S, Cepok S, Todorova-Rudolph A, *et al.* Etiology and site of temporal lobe epilepsy influence postictal cytokine release. Epilepsy Res 2009; 86(1): 82-8.
[http://dx.doi.org/10.1016/j.eplepsyres.2009.05.009] [PMID: 19520550]

[27]   Vezzani A, Ravizza T, Balosso S, Aronica E. Glia as a source of cytokines: implications for neuronal excitability and survival. Epilepsia 2008; 49 (Suppl. 2): 24-32.
[http://dx.doi.org/10.1111/j.1528-1167.2008.01490.x] [PMID: 18226169]

[28]   Nowell M, Miserocchi A, McEvoy AW, Duncan JS. Advances in epilepsy surgery. J Neurol Neurosurg Psychiatry 2014; 85(11): 1273-9.
[http://dx.doi.org/10.1136/jnnp-2013-307069] [PMID: 24719180]

[29]   Edwards CA, Kouzani A, Lee KH, Ross EK. Neurostimulation devices for the treatment of neurologic disorders. InMayo Clinic Proceedings 2017 Sep 1 (Vol. 92, No. 9, pp. 1427-1444). Elsevier.
[http://dx.doi.org/10.1016/j.mayocp.2017.05.005]

[30]   Ben-Menachem E. Vagus-nerve stimulation for the treatment of epilepsy. Lancet Neurol 2002; 1(8): 477-82.
[http://dx.doi.org/10.1016/S1474-4422(02)00220-X] [PMID: 12849332]

[31]   Bergey GK. Neurostimulation in the treatment of epilepsy. Exp Neurol 2013; 244: 87-95.
[http://dx.doi.org/10.1016/j.expneurol.2013.04.004] [PMID: 23583414]

[32]   Weinberg MS, McCown TJ. Current prospects and challenges for epilepsy gene therapy. Exp Neurol 2013; 244: 27-35.
[http://dx.doi.org/10.1016/j.expneurol.2011.10.003] [PMID: 22008258]

[33]   Simonato M. Gene therapy for epilepsy. Epilepsy Behav 2014; 38: 125-30.
[http://dx.doi.org/10.1016/j.yebeh.2013.09.013] [PMID: 24100249]

[34]   McCown TJ. Adeno-associated virus vector-mediated expression and constitutive secretion of galanin suppresses limbic seizure activity. Neurotherapeutics 2009; 6(2): 307-11.
[http://dx.doi.org/10.1016/j.nurt.2009.01.004] [PMID: 19332324]

[35]   Boison D. Adenosine kinase, epilepsy and stroke: mechanisms and therapies. Trends Pharmacol Sci 2006; 27(12): 652-8.
[http://dx.doi.org/10.1016/j.tips.2006.10.008] [PMID: 17056128]

[36]   Boison D, Stewart KA. Therapeutic epilepsy research: from pharmacological rationale to focal adenosine augmentation. Biochem Pharmacol 2009; 78(12): 1428-37.
[http://dx.doi.org/10.1016/j.bcp.2009.08.005] [PMID: 19682439]

[37]   Naegele JR, Maisano X, Yang J, Royston S, Ribeiro E. Recent advancements in stem cell and gene therapies for neurological disorders and intractable epilepsy. Neuropharmacology 2010; 58(6): 855-64.
[http://dx.doi.org/10.1016/j.neuropharm.2010.01.019] [PMID: 20146928]

[38]   Sørensen AT, Kokaia M. Novel approaches to epilepsy treatment. Epilepsia 2013; 54(1): 1-10.
[http://dx.doi.org/10.1111/epi.12000] [PMID: 23106744]

[39]   Wolff HG. Headache and other pain. 2nd Ed. New York: Oxford University Press; 1963. (3) "Definition: neuralgia". International Association for the Study of Pain taxonomy. Retrieved 5 August 2012.

[40]　Gilron I, Watson CP, Cahill CM, Moulin DE. Neuropathic pain: a practical guide for the clinician. CMAJ 2006; 175(3): 265-75.
[http://dx.doi.org/10.1503/cmaj.060146] [PMID: 16880448]

[41]　Medically reviewed by Beth Holloway. MD 2017; (April): 3.

[42]　Jensen TS. An improved understanding of neuropathic pain. Eur J Pain 2002; 6 (Suppl. B): 3-11.
[http://dx.doi.org/10.1016/S1090-3801(02)90002-9] [PMID: 23570142]

[43]　Benzon H, Rathmell JP, Wu CL, Turk D, Argoff CE, Hurley RW. Practical Management of Pain E-Book. Elsevier Health Sciences; 2013 Sep 11.

[44]　Zhu SM, Liu YM, An ED, Chen QL. Influence of systemic immune and cytokine responses during the acute phase of zoster on the development of postherpetic neuralgia. J Zhejiang Univ Sci B 2009; 10(8): 625-30.
[http://dx.doi.org/10.1631/jzus.B0920049] [PMID: 19650202]

[45]　Michael Stechison. Stechison, Michael Personal INTERVIEW 18 November 2008.

[46]　Daniel HC, Narewska J, Serpell M, Hoggart B, Johnson R, Rice AS. Comparison of psychological and physical function in neuropathic pain and nociceptive pain: implications for cognitive behavioral pain management programs. Eur J Pain 2008; 12(6): 731-41.
[http://dx.doi.org/10.1016/j.ejpain.2007.11.006] [PMID: 18164225]

[47]　Melzack R. The McGill Pain Questionnaire: major properties and scoring methods. Pain 1975; 1(3): 277-99.
[http://dx.doi.org/10.1016/0304-3959(75)90044-5] [PMID: 1235985]

[48]　Jensen TS. An improved understanding of neuropathic pain. Eur J Pain 2002; 6 (Suppl. B): 3-11.
[http://dx.doi.org/10.1016/S1090-3801(02)90002-9] [PMID: 23570142]

[49]　Garcia-Larrea L. Laser-evoked potentials in the diagnosis of central neuropathic pain. Douleur Analg 2008; 21(2): 93-8.
[http://dx.doi.org/10.1007/s11724-008-0092-5]

[50]　Rice AS, Maton S. Gabapentin in postherpetic neuralgia: a randomised, double blind, placebo controlled study. Pain 2001; 94(2): 215-24.
[http://dx.doi.org/10.1016/S0304-3959(01)00407-9] [PMID: 11690735]

[51]　Yang YJ, Hu L, Xia YP, *et al.* Resveratrol suppresses glial activation and alleviates trigeminal neuralgia *via* activation of AMPK. J Neuroinflammation 2016; 13(1): 84.
[http://dx.doi.org/10.1186/s12974-016-0550-6] [PMID: 27093858]

[52]　Schencking M, Sandholzer H, Frese T. Intravenous administration of vitamin C in the treatment of herpetic neuralgia: two case reports. Med Sci Monit 2010; 16(5): CS58-61.
[PMID: 20424557]

[53]　Tzabazis AZ, Klukinov M, Feliciano DP, Wilson SP, Yeomans DC. Gene therapy for trigeminal pain in mice. Gene Ther 2014; 21(4): 422-6.
[http://dx.doi.org/10.1038/gt.2014.14] [PMID: 24572785]

[54]　Matsushita Y, Araki K, Omotuyi Oi, Mukae T, Ueda H. HDAC inhibitors restore C-fibre sensitivity in experimental neuropathic pain model. Br J Pharmacol 2013; 170(5): 991-8.
[http://dx.doi.org/10.1111/bph.12366] [PMID: 24032674]

[55]　Denk F, Huang W, Sidders B, *et al.* HDAC inhibitors attenuate the development of hypersensitivity in models of neuropathic pain. Pain 2013; 154(9): 1668-79.
[http://dx.doi.org/10.1016/j.pain.2013.05.021] [PMID: 23693161]

[56]　Kiguchi N, Kobayashi Y, Maeda T, *et al.* Epigenetic augmentation of the macrophage inflammatory protein 2/C-X-C chemokine receptor type 2 axis through histone H3 acetylation in injured peripheral nerves elicits neuropathic pain. J Pharmacol Exp Ther 2012; 340(3): 577-87.
[http://dx.doi.org/10.1124/jpet.111.187724] [PMID: 22135382]

[57]   Zhu XY, Huang CS, Li Q, *et al.* p300 exerts an epigenetic role in chronic neuropathic pain through its acetyltransferase activity in rats following chronic constriction injury (CCI). Mol Pain 2012; 8: 84.
[http://dx.doi.org/10.1186/1744-8069-8-84] [PMID: 23176208]

[58]   Zhu X, Li Q, Chang R, *et al.* Curcumin alleviates neuropathic pain by inhibiting p300/CBP histone acetyltransferase activity-regulated expression of BDNF and cox-2 in a rat model. PLoS One 2014; 9(3)e91303
[http://dx.doi.org/10.1371/journal.pone.0091303] [PMID: 24603592]

[59]   Williams HL. Bell's palsy. AMA Arch Otolaryngol 1959; 70(4): 436-43.
[http://dx.doi.org/10.1001/archotol.1959.00730040446004] [PMID: 13844869]

[60]   Holland NJ, Weiner GM. Recent developments in Bell's palsy. BMJ 2004; 329(7465): 553-7.
[http://dx.doi.org/10.1136/bmj.329.7465.553] [PMID: 15345630]

[61]   Murakami S, Mizobuchi M, Nakashiro Y, Doi T, Hato N, Yanagihara N. Bell palsy and herpes simplex virus: identification of viral DNA in endoneurial fluid and muscle. Annals of internal medicine. 1996 Jan 1;124(1_Part_1):27-30.
[http://dx.doi.org/10.7326/0003-4819-124-1_Part_1-199601010-00005]

[62]   Zhang W, Xu L, Luo T, Wu F, Zhao B, Li X. The etiology of Bell's palsy: a review. J Neurol 2019; 1-0.
[http://dx.doi.org/10.1007/s00415-019-09282-4] [PMID: 30923934]

[63]   Yilmaz M, Tarakcıoğlu M, Bayazit N, Bayazit YA, Namiduru M, Kanlikama M. Serum cytokine levels in Bell's palsy. J Neurol Sci 2002; 197(1-2): 69-72.
[http://dx.doi.org/10.1016/S0022-510X(02)00049-7] [PMID: 11997069]

[64]   Baugh RF, Basura GJ, Ishii LE, *et al.* Clinical practice guideline: Bell's Palsy executive summary. Otolaryngol Head Neck Surg 2013; 149(5): 656-63.
[http://dx.doi.org/10.1177/0194599813506835] [PMID: 24190889]

[65]   Lorch M, Teach SJ. Facial nerve palsy: etiology and approach to diagnosis and treatment. Pediatr Emerg Care 2010; 26(10): 763-9.
[http://dx.doi.org/10.1097/PEC.0b013e3181f3bd4a] [PMID: 20930602]

[66]   Salinas RA, Alvarez G, Ferreira J. Corticosteroids for Bell's palsy (idiopathic facial paralysis). Cochrane database of systematic reviews. 2009(2).

[67]   Gagyor I, Madhok VB, Daly F, *et al.* Antiviral treatment for Bell's palsy (idiopathic facial paralysis). Cochrane Database of Systematic Reviews. 2015(9).

[68]   Hassoun HK. Role of Neurophysiology in predicting poor outcome in Bell's palsy. KUFA MEDICAL JOURNAL 2009; 12(2): 84-90.

[69]   Gantz BJ, Rubinstein JT, Gidley P, Woodworth GG. Surgical management of Bell's palsy. Laryngoscope 1999; 109(8): 1177-88.
[http://dx.doi.org/10.1097/00005537-199908000-00001] [PMID: 10443817]

[70]   "Syndrome Fact Sheet" NIAMS June 1, 2016 Archived from the original on 5 August 2016 Retrieved 13 August.

[71]   Carod-Artal FJ, Wichmann O, Farrar J, Gascón J. Neurological complications of dengue virus infection. Lancet Neurol 2013; 12(9): 906-19.
[http://dx.doi.org/10.1016/S1474-4422(13)70150-9] [PMID: 23948177]

[72]   Deresinski S, Monge-Maillo B, López-Vélez R, *et al.* Zika virus: a previously slow pandemic spreads rapidly through the Americas. Clin Infect Dis 2016; 62(5): iii-v.
[http://dx.doi.org/10.1093/cid/civ1009]

[73]   Ropper AH. The Guillain-Barré syndrome. N Engl J Med 1992; 326(17): 1130-6.
[http://dx.doi.org/10.1056/NEJM199204233261706] [PMID: 1552914]

[74]   Kuwabara S, Yuki N. Axonal Guillain-Barré syndrome: concepts and controversies. Lancet Neurol 2013; 12(12): 1180-8.
[http://dx.doi.org/10.1016/S1474-4422(13)70215-1] [PMID: 24229616]

[75]   Hohnoki K, Inoue A, Koh CS. Elevated serum levels of IFN-γ, IL-4 and TNF-α/unelevated serum levels of IL-10 in patients with demyelinating diseases during the acute stage. J Neuroimmunol 1998; 87(1-2): 27-32.
[http://dx.doi.org/10.1016/S0165-5728(98)00053-8] [PMID: 9670842]

[76]   Csurhes PA, Sullivan AA, Green K, Greer JM, Pender MP, McCombe PA. Increased circulating T cell reactivity to GM1 ganglioside in patients with Guillain-Barré syndrome. J Clin Neurosci 2005; 12(4): 409-15.
[http://dx.doi.org/10.1016/j.jocn.2004.04.006] [PMID: 15925771]

[77]   Elkarim RA, Dahle C, Mustafa M, *et al.* Recovery from Guillain-Barré syndrome is associated with increased levels of neutralizing autoantibodies to interferon-γ. Clin Immunol Immunopathol 1998; 88(3): 241-8.
[http://dx.doi.org/10.1006/clin.1998.4573] [PMID: 9743610]

[78]   Radhakrishnan VV, Sumi MG, Reuben S, Mathai A, Nair MD. Serum tumour necrosis factor-α and soluble tumour necrosis factor receptors levels in patients with Guillain-Barre syndrome. Acta Neurol Scand 2004; 109(1): 71-4.
[http://dx.doi.org/10.1034/j.1600-0404.2003.00179.x] [PMID: 14653854]

[79]   Kurz M, Pischel H, Hartung HP, Kieseier BC. Tumor necrosis factor-α-converting enzyme is expressed in the inflamed peripheral nervous system. J Peripher Nerv Syst 2005; 10(3): 311-8.
[http://dx.doi.org/10.1111/j.1085-9489.2005.10309.x] [PMID: 16221290]

[80]   Deng H, Yang X, Jin T, *et al.* The role of IL-12 and TNF-α in AIDP and AMAN. Eur J Neurol 2008; 15(10): 1100-5.
[http://dx.doi.org/10.1111/j.1468-1331.2008.02261.x] [PMID: 18717726]

[81]   Chen X, Bäumel M, Männel DN, Howard OM, Oppenheim JJ. Interaction of TNF with TNF receptor type 2 promotes expansion and function of mouse CD4+CD25+ T regulatory cells. J Immunol 2007; 179(1): 154-61.
[http://dx.doi.org/10.4049/jimmunol.179.1.154] [PMID: 17579033]

[82]   Hu W, Dehmel T, Pirhonen J, Hartung HP, Kieseier BC. Interleukin 23 in acute inflammatory demyelination of the peripheral nerve. Arch Neurol 2006; 63(6): 858-64.
[http://dx.doi.org/10.1001/archneur.63.6.858] [PMID: 16769867]

[83]   Sivieri S, Ferrarini AM, Lolli F, *et al.* Cytokine pattern in the cerebrospinal fluid from patients with GBS and CIDP. J Neurol Sci 1997; 147(1): 93-5.
[http://dx.doi.org/10.1016/S0022-510X(96)00319-X] [PMID: 9094066]

[84]   Hayashi R, Xiao W, Kawamoto M, Yuge O, Bennett GJ. Systemic glucocorticoid therapy reduces pain and the number of endoneurial tumor necrosis factor-alpha (TNFα)-positive mast cells in rats with a painful peripheral neuropathy. J Pharmacol Sci 2008; •••0804020090
[http://dx.doi.org/10.1254/jphs.FP0072181]

[85]   Jander S, Stoll G. Interleukin-18 is induced in acute inflammatory demyelinating polyneuropathy. J Neuroimmunol 2001; 114(1-2): 253-8.
[http://dx.doi.org/10.1016/S0165-5728(00)00460-4] [PMID: 11240039]

[86]   Zhu J, Link H, Weerth S, Linington C, Mix E, Qiao J. The B cell repertoire in experimental allergic neuritis involves multiple myelin proteins and GM1. J Neurol Sci 1994; 125(2): 132-7.
[http://dx.doi.org/10.1016/0022-510X(94)90025-6] [PMID: 7528788]

[87]   Weller M, Stevens A, Sommer N, Melms A, Dichgans J, Wiethölter H. Comparative analysis of cytokine patterns in immunological, infectious, and oncological neurological disorders. J Neurol Sci 1991; 104(2): 215-21.

[http://dx.doi.org/10.1016/0022-510X(91)90313-V] [PMID: 1940975]

[88]   Ossege LM, Sindern E, Voss B, Malin JP. Expression of TNFalpha and TGFbeta1 in Guillain-Barré syndrome: correlation of a low TNFalpha-/TGFbeta1-mRNA ratio with good recovery and signs for immunoregulation within the cerebrospinal fluid compartment. Eur J Neurol 2000; 7(1): 17-25.
[http://dx.doi.org/10.1046/j.1468-1331.2000.00005.x] [PMID: 10809911]

[89]   Press R, Ozenci V, Kouwenhoven M, Link H. Non-T(H)1 cytokines are augmented systematically early in Guillain-Barré syndrome. Neurology 2002; 58(3): 476-8.
[http://dx.doi.org/10.1212/WNL.58.3.476] [PMID: 11839856]

[90]   Lu MO, Zhu J. The role of cytokines in Guillain-Barré syndrome. J Neurol 2011; 258(4): 533-48.
[http://dx.doi.org/10.1007/s00415-010-5836-5] [PMID: 21104265]

[91]   Dahle C, Ekerfelt C, Vrethem M, Samuelsson M, Ernerudh J. T helper type 2 like cytokine responses to peptides from P0 and P2 myelin proteins during the recovery phase of Guillain-Barré syndrome. J Neurol Sci 1997; 153(1): 54-60.
[http://dx.doi.org/10.1016/S0022-510X(97)00178-0] [PMID: 9455979]

[92]   Press R, Pashenkov M, Jin JP, Link H. Aberrated levels of cerebrospinal fluid chemokines in Guillain-Barré syndrome and chronic inflammatory demyelinating polyradiculoneuropathy. J Clin Immunol 2003; 23(4): 259-67.
[http://dx.doi.org/10.1023/A:1024532715775] [PMID: 12959218]

[93]   van den Berg B, Walgaard C, Drenthen J, Fokke C, Jacobs BC, van Doorn PA. Guillain-Barré syndrome: pathogenesis, diagnosis, treatment and prognosis. Nat Rev Neurol 2014; 10(8): 469-82.
[http://dx.doi.org/10.1038/nrneurol.2014.121] [PMID: 25023340]

[94]   Eldar AH, Chapman J. Guillain Barré syndrome and other immune mediated neuropathies: diagnosis and classification. Autoimmun Rev 2014; 13(4-5): 525-30.
[http://dx.doi.org/10.1016/j.autrev.2014.01.033] [PMID: 24434363]

[95]   Spasovski G, Vanholder R, Allolio B, *et al.* Clinical practice guideline on diagnosis and treatment of hyponatraemia. Nephrology Dialysis Transplantation. 2014 Apr 1;29(suppl_2):i1-39.

[96]   Hughes RA, Swan AV, Raphaël JC, Annane D, van Koningsveld R, van Doorn PA. Immunotherapy for Guillain-Barré syndrome: a systematic review. Brain 2007; 130(Pt 9): 2245-57.
[http://dx.doi.org/10.1093/brain/awm004] [PMID: 17337484]

[97]   Dimachkie MM, Barohn RJ. Guillain-Barré syndrome and variants. Neurol Clin 2013; 31(2): 491-510.
[http://dx.doi.org/10.1016/j.ncl.2013.01.005] [PMID: 23642721]

[98]   https://forum.gbs-cidp.org/forums/topic/stem-cell-treatment/#post-3652

[99]   Potential treatment target for Guillain-Barré syndrome www.sciencedaily.com/releases/2016/08/160823102236.htm

[100]   Chitnis T, Najafian N, Benou C, *et al.* Effect of targeted disruption of STAT4 and STAT6 on the induction of experimental autoimmune encephalomyelitis. J Clin Invest 2001; 108(5): 739-47.
[http://dx.doi.org/10.1172/JCI200112563] [PMID: 11544280]

[101]   Wurster AL, Tanaka T, Grusby MJ. The biology of Stat4 and Stat6. Oncogene 2000; 19(21): 2577-84.
[http://dx.doi.org/10.1038/sj.onc.1203485] [PMID: 10851056]

[102]   Kaplan MH, Sun YL, Hoey T, Grusby MJ. Impaired IL-12 responses and enhanced development of Th2 cells in Stat4-deficient mice. Nature 1996; 382(6587): 174-7.
[http://dx.doi.org/10.1038/382174a0] [PMID: 8700209]

[103]   Roman-Blas JA, Jimenez SA. Targeting NF-kappaB: a promising molecular therapy in inflammatory arthritis. Int Rev Immunol 2008; 27(5): 351-74.
[http://dx.doi.org/10.1080/08830180802295740] [PMID: 18853343]

[104]   Brereton CF, Sutton CE, Lalor SJ, Lavelle EC, Mills KH. Inhibition of ERK MAPK suppresses IL-23- and IL-1-driven IL-17 production and attenuates autoimmune disease. J Immunol 2009; 183(3): 1715-

23.
[http://dx.doi.org/10.4049/jimmunol.0803851] [PMID: 19570828]

[105]　Wu T, Mohan C. The AKT axis as a therapeutic target in autoimmune diseases. Endocrine, Metabolic & Immune Disorders-Drug Targets (Formerly Current Drug Targets-Immune, Endocrine & Metabolic Disorders). 2009 Jun 1;9(2):145-50.
[http://dx.doi.org/10.2174/187153009788452417]

[106]　Peifer C, Wagner G, Laufer S. New approaches to the treatment of inflammatory disorders small molecule inhibitors of p38 MAP kinase. Curr Top Med Chem 2006; 6(2): 113-49.
[http://dx.doi.org/10.2174/156802606775270323] [PMID: 16454763]

[107]　Ding C, Xu J, Li J. ABT-874, a fully human monoclonal anti-IL-12/IL-23 antibody for the potential treatment of autoimmune diseases. Curr Opin Investig Drugs 2008; 9(5): 515-22.
[PMID: 18465662]

[108]　Billich A. Drug evaluation: apilimod, an oral IL-12/IL-23 inhibitor for the treatment of autoimmune diseases and common variable immunodeficiency. IDrugs: the investigational drugs journal. 2007 Jan;10(1):53-9.

[109]　Wittig BM. Drug evaluation: CNTO-1275, a mAb against IL-12/IL-23p40 for the potential treatment of inflammatory diseases. Current opinion in investigational drugs (London, England: 2000). 2007 Nov;8(11):947-54.

[110]　Skurkovich S, Boiko A, Beliaeva I, *et al.* Randomized study of antibodies to IFN-gamma and TNF-alpha in secondary progressive multiple sclerosis. Mult Scler 2001; 7(5): 277-84.
[PMID: 11724442]

[111]　Csurhes PA, Sullivan AA, Green K, Pender MP, McCombe PA. T cell reactivity to P0, P2, PMP-22, and myelin basic protein in patients with Guillain-Barre syndrome and chronic inflammatory demyelinating polyradiculoneuropathy. J Neurol Neurosurg Psychiatry 2005; 76(10): 1431-9.
[http://dx.doi.org/10.1136/jnnp.2004.052282] [PMID: 16170091]

[112]　Saver JL, Warach S, Janis S, *et al.* Standardizing the structure of stroke clinical and epidemiologic research data: the National Institute of Neurological Disorders and Stroke (NINDS) Stroke Common Data Element (CDE) project. Stroke 2012; 43(4): 967-73.
[http://dx.doi.org/10.1161/STROKEAHA.111.634352] [PMID: 22308239]

[113]　Dayalu P, Albin RL. Huntington disease: pathogenesis and treatment. Neurol Clin 2015; 33(1): 101-14.
[http://dx.doi.org/10.1016/j.ncl.2014.09.003] [PMID: 25432725]

[114]　Shcherbinina M. PSY 3130.

[115]　Frank S. Treatment of Huntington's disease. Neurotherapeutics 2014; 11(1): 153-60.
[http://dx.doi.org/10.1007/s13311-013-0244-z] [PMID: 24366610]

[116]　Purves D, Augustine GJ, Fitzpatrick D, *et al.* Circuits within the basal ganglia system InNeuroscience. 2nd ed., Sinauer Associates 2001.

[117]　Liu Z, Zhou T, Ziegler AC, Dimitrion P, Zuo L. Oxidative stress in neurodegenerative diseases: from molecular mechanisms to clinical applications. Oxidative medicine and cellular longevity. 2017; 2017.
[http://dx.doi.org/10.1155/2017/2525967]

[118]　Crossman AR. Functional anatomy of movement disorders. J Anat 2000; 196(Pt 4): 519-25.
[http://dx.doi.org/10.1046/j.1469-7580.2000.19640519.x] [PMID: 10923984]

[119]　Duffy JR. Motor speech disorders: Substrates, differential diagnosis, and management: Elsevier Health Sciences. 2012.

[120]　Hersch SM, Gevorkian S, Marder K, *et al.* Creatine in Huntington disease is safe, tolerable, bioavailable in brain and reduces serum 8OH2'dG. Neurology 2006; 66(2): 250-2.
[http://dx.doi.org/10.1212/01.wnl.0000194318.74946.b6] [PMID: 16434666]

[121] Suh JH, Wang H, Liu RM, Liu J, Hagen TM. (R)-α-lipoic acid reverses the age-related loss in GSH redox status in post-mitotic tissues: evidence for increased cysteine requirement for GSH synthesis. Arch Biochem Biophys 2004; 423(1): 126-35.
[http://dx.doi.org/10.1016/j.abb.2003.12.020] [PMID: 14871476]

[122] Shenk JC, Liu J, Fischbach K, *et al.* The effect of acetyl-L-carnitine and R-α-lipoic acid treatment in ApoE4 mouse as a model of human Alzheimer's disease. J Neurol Sci 2009; 283(1-2): 199-206.
[http://dx.doi.org/10.1016/j.jns.2009.03.002] [PMID: 19342064]

[123] Dunnett SB, Rosser AE. Cell therapy in Huntington's disease. NeuroRx 2004; 1(4): 394-405.
[http://dx.doi.org/10.1602/neurorx.1.4.394] [PMID: 15717043]

[124] Sanberg PR, Borlongan CV, Wictorin K, Isacson O. Fetal-Tissue Transplantation for Huntington's Disease: Preclinical Studies InCell Transplantation for Neurological Disorders. Totowa, NJ: Humana Press 1998; pp. 77-93.

[125] Bosch M, Pineda JR, Suñol C, *et al.* Induction of GABAergic phenotype in a neural stem cell line for transplantation in an excitotoxic model of Huntington's disease. Exp Neurol 2004; 190(1): 42-58.
[http://dx.doi.org/10.1016/j.expneurol.2004.06.027] [PMID: 15473979]

[126] DiFiglia M. Excitotoxic injury of the neostriatum: a model for Huntington's disease. Trends Neurosci 1990; 13(7): 286-9.
[http://dx.doi.org/10.1016/0166-2236(90)90111-M] [PMID: 1695405]

[127] Kim M, Lee ST, Chu K, Kim SU. Stem cell-based cell therapy for Huntington disease: a review. Neuropathology 2008; 28(1): 1-9.
[http://dx.doi.org/10.1111/j.1440-1789.2007.00858.x] [PMID: 18069970]

[128] Šramka M, Rattaj M, Molina H, Vojtassák J, Belan V, Ruzický E. Stereotactic technique and pathophysiological mechanisms of neurotransplantation in Huntington's chorea. Stereotact Funct Neurosurg 1992; 58(1-4): 79-83.
[http://dx.doi.org/10.1159/000098976] [PMID: 1439353]

[129] Kopyov OV, Jacques S, Kurth M, *et al.* Fetal transplantation for Huntington's disease: clinical studies InCell transplantation for neurological disorders. Totowa, NJ: Humana Press 1998; pp. 95-134.

[130] Vonsattel JP, DiFiglia M. Huntington disease. J Neuropathol Exp Neurol 1998; 57(5): 369-84.
[http://dx.doi.org/10.1097/00005072-199805000-00001] [PMID: 9596408]

[131] Ferrante RJ, Kowall NW, Beal MF, Richardson EP Jr, Bird ED, Martin JB. Selective sparing of a class of striatal neurons in Huntington's disease. Science 1985; 230(4725): 561-3.
[http://dx.doi.org/10.1126/science.2931802] [PMID: 2931802]

[132] Ryu JK, Kim J, Cho SJ, *et al.* Proactive transplantation of human neural stem cells prevents degeneration of striatal neurons in a rat model of Huntington disease. Neurobiol Dis 2004; 16(1): 68-77.
[http://dx.doi.org/10.1016/j.nbd.2004.01.016] [PMID: 15207263]

[133] Kordower JH, Chen EY, Winkler C, *et al.* Grafts of EGF-responsive neural stem cells derived from GFAP-hNGF transgenic mice: trophic and tropic effects in a rodent model of Huntington's disease. J Comp Neurol 1997; 387(1): 96-113.
[http://dx.doi.org/10.1002/(SICI)1096-9861(19971013)387:1<96::AID-CNE8>3.0.CO;2-I] [PMID: 9331174]

[134] Roberts TJ, Price J, Williams SC, Modo M. Preservation of striatal tissue and behavioral function after neural stem cell transplantation in a rat model of Huntington's disease. Neuroscience 2006; 139(4): 1187-99.
[http://dx.doi.org/10.1016/j.neuroscience.2006.01.025] [PMID: 16517087]

[135] Lescaudron L, Unni D, Dunbar GL. Autologous adult bone marrow stem cell transplantation in an animal model of huntington's disease: behavioral and morphological outcomes. Int J Neurosci 2003; 113(7): 945-56.

[http://dx.doi.org/10.1080/00207450390207759] [PMID: 12881187]

[136] Schmidt NO, Przylecki W, Yang W, *et al.* Brain tumor tropism of transplanted human neural stem cells is induced by vascular endothelial growth factor. Neoplasia 2005; 7(6): 623-9.
[http://dx.doi.org/10.1593/neo.04781] [PMID: 16036113]

[137] Sun L, Lee J, Fine HA. Neuronally expressed stem cell factor induces neural stem cell migration to areas of brain injury. J Clin Invest 2004; 113(9): 1364-74.
[http://dx.doi.org/10.1172/JCI200420001] [PMID: 15124028]

[138] Ehtesham M, Yuan X, Kabos P, *et al.* Glioma tropic neural stem cells consist of astrocytic precursors and their migratory capacity is mediated by CXCR4. Neoplasia 2004; 6(3): 287-93.
[http://dx.doi.org/10.1593/neo.03427] [PMID: 15153341]

[139] Steffan JS, Bodai L, Pallos J, *et al.* Histone deacetylase inhibitors arrest polyglutamine-dependent neurodegeneration in Drosophila. Nature 2001; 413(6857): 739-43.
[http://dx.doi.org/10.1038/35099568] [PMID: 11607033]

[140] Lim RG, Salazar LL, Wilton DK, *et al.* Developmental alterations in Huntington's disease neural cells and pharmacological rescue in cells and mice. Nat Neurosci 2017; 20(5): 648-60.
[http://dx.doi.org/10.1038/nn.4532] [PMID: 28319609]

[141] Lee J, Hwang YJ, Kim Y, *et al.* Remodeling of heterochromatin structure slows neuropathological progression and prolongs survival in an animal model of Huntington's disease. Acta Neuropathol 2017; 134(5): 729-48.
[http://dx.doi.org/10.1007/s00401-017-1732-8] [PMID: 28593442]

[142] Guo X, Disatnik MH, Monbureau M, Shamloo M, Mochly-Rosen D, Qi X. Inhibition of mitochondrial fragmentation diminishes Huntington's disease-associated neurodegeneration. J Clin Invest 2013; 123(12): 5371-88.
[http://dx.doi.org/10.1172/JCI70911] [PMID: 24231356]

CHAPTER 4

Screening Models For Neuroleptic Drug-Induced Hyperprolactinemia: A Mini-Review

Prashant Tiwari[1,*], Sunil Kumar Dubey[2], Shweta Shrivastava[1] and Pratap Kumar Sahu[3]

[1] *School of Pharmacy, School of Health and Allied Sciences, ARKA JAIN University, Jamshedpur - 832102, India*

[2] *Institute of Pharmacy, Birla Institute of Technology and Science, Pilani, Rajasthan - 333031, India*

[3] *Department of Pharmacology, School of Pharmaceutical Sciences, Siksha O Anusandhan (Deemed to be University), Bhubaneswar - 751029, India*

Abstract: Schizophrenia is a thought disorder characterized by hallucinations, delusions, and disorganized thinking. It affects 1% of the world population. Neuroleptics are the drugs used in the treatment of schizophrenia. Besides extrapyramidal side effects, hyperprolactinemia is a major side effect with neuroleptics like haloperidol, risperidone, *etc*. Hyperprolactinemia results in gynecomastia (male), galactorrhoea, oligomenorrhoea, and amenorrhoea (female) which leads to sexual dysfunction and infertility. Dopamine receptor agonists like cabergoline, bromocriptine, *etc* are used in the treatment of hyperprolactinemia. However, these drugs may aggravate the symptoms of schizophrenia. So, there is a need for the discovery of drugs that can be used against neuroleptic drug-induced hyperprolactinemia. Lack of suitable animal models for the evaluation of new drugs against neuroleptic drug-induced hyperprolactinemia is a major concern. In this chapter, reviews on neuroleptic drug-induced hyperprolactinemia and the available animal models for the screening of hyperprolactinemia are included.

Keywords: Animal Model, Hyperprolactinemia, Neuroleptic, Schizophrenia.

INTRODUCTION

Schizophrenia is a thought disorder characterized by unusual behavior and the inability to understand and accept the truth. **People with schizophrenia also experience other mental disorders** such as anxiety, depression, *etc.* [1 - 4]. Its symptoms include positive symptoms (delusions, hallucinations), negative symptoms (withdrawal from society, flattening of emotional response), cognitive

---

[*] **Corresponding author Prashant Tiwari**: School of Pharmacy, School of Health and Allied Sciences, ARKA JAIN University, Jamshedpur, India; Tel: +91-7828865022; E mail:dr.prashant@arkajainuniversity.ac.in

Atta-ur-Rahman & Zareen Amtul (Eds.)

All rights reserved-© 2020 Bentham Science Publishers

impairments, and affective dysregulation [5 - 7]. The prevalence of schizophrenia is about 1% of the world population. Americans show a high prevalence of around 1.2% [8].

The drugs used to control schizophrenia are antipsychotics or neuroleptics or major tranquilizers [9]. Positive symptoms respond well to conventional antipsychotic medications. However, negative symptoms and cognitive impairments show a negligible response towards antipsychotics [5 - 7]. First-generation antipsychotics are also known as typical antipsychotics. They came into insight and use in the 1950s. Few examples are chlorpromazine, haloperidol, *etc*. They act by blocking dopamine (D2) receptors. Second-generation drugs are known as atypical antipsychotics. The first atypical antipsychotic, clozapine, was discovered in the 1960s and introduced clinically in the 1970s [10]. They act by blocking serotonin receptors in addition to dopamine receptors [11].

Antipsychotic drugs are associated with a range of side effects in most patients. The most troublesome side effects are neurologically known as extrapyramidal side effects (EPS). The typical antipsychotics are more associated with EPS which includes drug-induced Parkinsonism, akathisia, and tardive dyskinesia, *etc*. The atypical antipsychotics show fewer EPS while producing an increased risk of agranulocytosis, seizures, and weight gain1 [2 - 14].

However, both typical, as well as atypical antipsychotics, increases prolactin levels by 10-fold or more than pretreatment values. Approximately 60% of women and 40% of men treated with a prolactin-raising antipsychotic had a prolactin level above the upper limit of the normal range. Hyperprolactinemia results in gynecomastia (male), galactorrhoea, oligomenorrhoea, and amenorrhoea (female) which leads to sexual dysfunction and infertility [15 - 17].

PROLACTIN

Prolactin is a lactogenic hormone secreted from the pituitary gland in the brain. The main action of prolactin is to maintain lactation through which there is a stimulation of the mammary gland to secrete milk. When prolactin serum concentration increased during pregnancy causes enlargement of mammary glands, then milk production starts. It happens because of a decrease in the progesterone level during pregnancy [18]. Prolactin has a key role in the regulation of the immune system, pancreatic development, affects adipose tissue, and the body metabolism [19]. The secretion of the prolactin hormone is managed by endocrine neurons at the base of the forebrain. Prolactin is regulated by dopamine. Elevated serum prolactin levels can cause an irregular menstrual cycle and galactorrhoea in females [20, 21].

Prolactin Receptor

Prolactin is a member of class 1 cytokine receptors. Prolactin receptor has a wide tissue distribution including mammary glands, uterus, placenta, adrenal gland, gonads as well as liver, kidney, heart, lung, skin, lymphoid cells, and brain. Prolactin receptor is a tyrosine kinase linked receptor. Prolactin acts as a cytokine. Different actions have been reported for prolactin in various tissues. Human prolactin is present on chromosome 5 and consists of nine coding exons and two noncoding exons [22]. However, regulation of prolactin levels occurs at transcription and post-transcriptional levels. It has come into notice that prolactin degradation may be helpful for the inhibition of breast cell transformation [23, 24]. Further, binding of prolactin receptor may cause dimerization with [BPB1] another prolactin receptor which leads to activate non-receptor tyrosine kinase that recruits the Janus kinase, single transducer and activators of transcription proteins which ultimately activates mitogen-activated protein kinase (MAPK) and Src kinase. This results in the activation of Janus kinase 2, a tyrosine kinase that initiates the JAK-STAT pathway which ultimately activates mitogen-activated protein kinase (MAPK) and Src kinase [25 - 27].

Normal Prolactin Level

The prolactin level is measured in nanograms per milliliter (ng/mL). Normal levels in human beings are: females- less than 25 ng/mL, males- less than 17 ng/mL [28]. Serum prolactin level is sometimes given as nanomole per liter [29]. The normal serum prolactin levels in men and women vary between <20 µg/L and <25 µg/L. The normal plasma level in male rats are 8 to 33 ng/mL and female rats is 43 to 977 ng/mL [30].

HYPERPROLACTINEMIA

Hyperprolactinemia is a condition of elevated serum prolactin [31]. Pituitary Society (PS) suggested that PRL values up to 100 mg/L (2000 mU/L) may be due to antipsychotic drugs, whereas macroprolactinomas are typically associated with levels >25 mg/L (>5000 mg/L) [32]. Moreover, PRL level in non-functioning pituitary adenomas is almost always <100 mg/L (<2000 mg/L) [29]. Pituitary tumors account for 50% of cases of hyperprolactinemia which seeks its proper investigation in the absence of drug-induced hyperprolactinemia [33, 34].

Drug-Induced Hyperprolactinemia

Neuroleptic drug use is a common and severe cause of hyperprolactinemia. Disturbance in prolactin levels is one of the most common endocrine disorders [35]. However, some of the pathological causes such as prolactin associated pituitary tumors is accountable for elevated serum prolactin levels. There are a number of antipsychotics drugs like alprazolam, moclobemide, amitriptyline, haloperidol, Compazine, risperidone, chlorpromazine, perphenazine, sulpiride, metoclopramide, *etc* is responsible for increased serum prolactin level [36]. Drugs that are the most common cause of hyperprolactinemia are listed in Table (**1** and **2**). When serum prolactin levels elevated, there is an immediate need to discontinue the treatment until the prolactin level return to its normal value [37, 38]. Hyperprolactinemia causes inhibition of the hypothalamus secretion of gonadotropin-releasing hormone which in turn results in the release of gonads sex hormone by inhibiting the release of follicle-stimulating hormone (FSH) and luteinizing hormone (LH) [39 - 43].

Table 1. Causative agents for hyperprolactinemia[15].

Antipsychotics	Typical	Atypical
	Haloperidol Chlorpromazine, Thioridazine, Thiothixene	Risperidone, Amisulpride Molindone, Zotepine
	Typical Antipsychotics Phenothiazines: Chlorpromazine, Fluphenazine, Thioridazine Butyrophenones: Haloperidol, Droperidol, Penfluridol, Trifluperidol. Thioxanthene: Flupenthixol, Chlorprothixene, Cyclopethanol, Thiothixene **Atypical Antipsychotics** Dibenzothiazepines:Clozapine, Olanzapine Dibenzoxazepine: Loxapine Dihydroindolone:Molindone Diphenyl Butylpyridine:Pimozide, Penfluridol Benzamide:Sulpiride Benzisoxazole:Risperidone	

Clinical Hyperprolactinemia

Hyperprolactinemia is reported in schizophrenic patients taking neuroleptic drugs. Risperidone 10 mg/day for a period of 8 weeks showed a significant increase in serum prolactin levels [48, 49]. Risperidone and clozapine-induced hyperprolactinemia in outpatients with schizophrenia [50]. Sulpiride 150mg/day for 10 days sulpiride causes hyperprolactinemia. Amisulpride (50–800 mg/day for 13to 50 days) was found to significantly increase plasma prolactin [51]. Similar results were observed in Korean patients when treated with 300 mg/day of amisulpride [52]. Levosulpiride also develops serum prolactin levels of > 200 ng/mL [53]. Patients receiving haloperidol at a dose of 10-20 mg for a period of 60 weeks showed a significant increase in prolactin concentration (30 and 50 ng/ml).In another study, Olanzapine moderately elevates PRL *i.e.* 1-4 ng/ml, haloperidol significantly increased PRL *i.e.* 17 ng/ml whereas, risperidone strongly increase PRL *i.e.* 45-80 ng/ml [54].

Table 2. Causes of Hyperprolactinemia [44 - 47].

Physiologic hypersecretion	Coitus, Pregnancy, Lactation, Chest wall stimulation Sleep, Stress, Lunch or Dinner, Lactation, and Mammary stimulus.
Pathological hypersecretion	Infiltrative disorders, Non-functioning pituitary tumors, Empty sella syndrome, Hypothyroidism, and during renal failure.
Pituitary hypersecretion	Prolactinoma, Acromegaly and Laron syndrome.
Pituitary diseases	Functioning adenomas, Non-functioning adenomas, and Abnormal stalk.
Hypothalamic-pituitary stalk damage	Craniopharyngioma, Irradiation, Inflammation, Trauma and Suprasellar surgery.
Systemic disorders	Hypothyroidism, Cranial radiation.

Treatment of Hyperprolactinemia

Dopamine agonist like bromocriptine is the choice of treatment for hyperprolactinemia. These drugs decrease serum prolactin concentrations and decrease the size of most lactotroph adenomas [55]. Generally, cabergoline is the drug of the second choice but in some, cases cabergoline is the unlike preferable drug due to its safety and efficacy than bromocriptine (cause nausea like cabergoline) [56 - 61].

Quinagolide (CV 205-502) is a non-ergot dopamine agonist [62 - 64]. Quinagolide works in a similar way towards decreasing the serum prolactin level and adenoma size as cabergoline [64]. The development of key side effects in patients such as postural hypotension, nausea, mental fogginess which are witnessed with the use of dopamine agonist drug can be prevented by the use of its small dose of haloperidol (1, 2, and 5 mg/kg/day)and sulpiride (20 and 40 mg/kg/day) and administering it with food or during bedtime [65, 66].

Neuroleptic drug-induced hyperprolactinemia can also be countered by use of dopamine agonists. However, this may lead to compromising the efficacy of neuroleptics because of the role of dopamine in the pathophysiology of schizophrenia [67]. So, there is a need to develop drugs for neuroleptic drug-induced hyperprolactinemia which should not affect dopaminergic function as a neurotransmitters released by neuronal cells to send a signals to other nerve cells.The brain includes several distinct dopamine pathways, one of which plays a major role in the motivational component of reward-motivated behavior. Screening with animal models is the first step in the drug discovery process [68]. As per available literature few animal models are available to evaluate hyperprolactinemia produced by neuroleptic drugs. These animal models have many limitations.

There is a contradiction about specific dose, timing, duration, and selection of animals either male or female. Few available preclinical models of drug-induced hyperprolactinemia are discussed here.

PRE-CLINICAL SCREENING MODELS FOR HYPERPROLACTINEMIA

Most animal models of hyperprolactinemia use antipsychotic drugs. Hyperprolactinemia can also be induced by metoclopramide and prolactin. The various pre-clinical animal models for screening of hyperprolactinemia have been tabulated in brief in Table **3**.

Prolactin Model

Rehman *et al*, injected 5 mg rat prolactin subcutaneously (SQ) daily for 1 week in two divided doses for induction of hyperprolactinemia and they found an elevated level of prolactin (500 ng/ml) in the treated group as compared to control (20 ng/ml) [69].

Haloperidol (HPL) Model

Savita *et al* showed that intraperitoneal administration of haloperidol for 16 days at doses level (1, 2 and 5 mg/kg/day) significantly produced hyperprolactinemia in female albino rats. The drugs were administered once daily. On the 17th day, all animals were sacrificed and blood was drawn from the tail vein for measurement of PRL [70, 71]. This study has a limitation that only female rats were used and they have not specified the optimal dose level for induction of hyperprolactinemia caused by haloperidol. Again, out of the three doses, they should have suggested (5 mg/kg/day) dose. We have induced hyperprolactinemia using haloperidol 5 mg/kg/day for 16 days and successfully evaluated effect of *Butea monosperma* (200 mg/kg/day/p.o. and 400 mg/kg/day/p.o.) and *Tinospora cordifolia* (200 mg/kg/day/p.o. and 400 mg/kg/day/p.o.) on hyperprolactinemia [72, 73].

Metoclopramide (MCP) Model

Metoclopramide (MCP) (24 mg/kg thrice daily for 5 days, 75 mg/kg twice daily for 15 days and 150 mg/kg daily for 10 days i.p.) can be used as a screening model to induce hyperprolactinemia [55, 74]. Several studies used different doses and different durations. The albino rats were given intraperitoneally MCP 150 mg/kg daily, for 10 days. Thereafter at the day 14, blood was drawn from the tail vein for the measurement of PRL. It was observed that at least 80% elevation of serum PRL concentrations was found in the drug-treated group as compared to the control group [75]. Intraperitoneal injection of MCP (75 mg/kg, twice daily) was given for 15 days to albino rats, and on the 15th day after the treatment, the blood sample was collected from the orbit vein. It was noticed that there was a significant increase in serum PRL levels [76]. Hyperprolactinemia was induced after the daily administration of metoclopramide dihydrochloride (24 mg/kg body wt., 3 times a day) for 5 days. The levels of the serum prolactin were significantly greater (p<0.01) than normal animals. In addition, for the evaluation of serum prolactin level, the albino mice were used for the study [77]. One study also used estrogen and progesterone in addition to MCP to induce hyperprolactinemia. Metoclopramide hydrochloride injection (50 mg/kg) was administered for 5 days. After that estradiol was injected for twenty-five days then progesterone was administered for five days and at the end, the PRL in Wistar rats' serum were measured and there was hyperprolactinemia [78].

Sulpiride Model

Administration of sulpiride at a dose of 20 mg/kg intraperitoneally for a period of 28 days in rats showed a remarkable rise in PRL [79]. Similarly, administration of sulpiride daily intraperitoneally at a dose of 40 mg/kg in male Wistar rats for 30 and 60 days significantly increases plasma PRL levels [80]. We have induced hyperprolactinemia using sulpiride 20 mg/kg/day for 28 days and successfully evaluated effect of the *Butea monosperma* (200 mg/kg/day/p.o. and 400 mg/kg/day/p.o.) and *Tinospora cordifolia* (200 mg/kg/day/p.o. and 400 mg/kg/day/p.o.) on hyperprolactinemia [72, 73].

MANAGEMENT OF HYPERPROLACTINEMIA

Dopamine agonist like bromocriptine is the choice of treatment for hyperprolactinemia. These drugs decrease serum prolactin concentrations and decrease the size of most lactotroph adenomas [81]. Cabergoline is the drug of the first choice as it is safe and efficacious. Bromocriptine is the drug of second choice [82 - 86]. Bromocriptine is an ergot derivative. It is more likely to cause nausea than cabergoline [87].

Quinagolide (CV 205-502) is a non-ergot dopamine agonist [88, 89]. Quinagolide works in a similar way towards decreasing the serum prolactin level and adenoma size as cabergoline [90]. The development of key side effects in patients such as postural hypotension, nausea, mental fogginess which are witnessed with the use of dopamine agonist drugs can be prevented by the use of its small dose and administering it with food or during bedtime [91, 92].

Neuroleptic drug-induced hyperprolactinemia can also be countered by use of dopamine agonists. However, this may lead to compromising the efficacy of neuroleptics because of the impact of dopamine in the pathophysiology of schizophrenia [93]. So, there is a need to develop drugs for neuroleptic drug-induced hyperprolactinemia which should not affect dopaminergic function. Screening with animal models is the first step in the drug discovery process [94].

Table 3. Animal models for pre-clinical screening study [69 - 80].

Animal Model	Drug	Dose	Rout of Drug Administration	Duration
Albino Rats	Prolactin	5 mg/kg/day	Subcutaneous (sq.)	1 week
Albino Rats	Haloperidol	1, 2 & 5 mg/kg/day	Intraperitonial (i.p)	16 days
Albino Mice	Metoclopramide	24 mg/kg	Intraperitonial (i.p)	Thrice daily for 5 days
Albino Rats	Metoclopramide	75 mg/kg	Intraperitonial (i.p)	Twice daily for 15 days
Albino Rats	Metoclopramide	150 mg/kg/day	Intraperitonial (i.p)	10 days
Wistar rats	Metoclopramide	50 mg/kg/day	Intraperitonial (i.p)	5 days
Wistar rats	Sulpiride	20, 40 mg/kg/day	Intraperitonial (i.p)	28 days
Wistar rats	Sulpiride	20, 40 mg/kg/day	Intraperitonial (i.p)	30 & 60 days

Surgical Treatment of Prolactin

There are limited dopaminergic drugs available to subside the adverse event of neuroleptic drugs. Currently, dopaminergic drugs are the choice of treatment for the symptoms of prolactin, but presently hyperprolactinemic symptoms can also be reduced by the surgery. However, the success rate of clinical surgery is very poor and even sometimes very critical to operating the prolactinoma patients. Moreover, some of the studies revealed that now a days hyperprolactinemia may occur within four years after the surgery. One of the studies suggested that transsphenoidal surgery (TS) may be proposed as conclusive therapy. This therapy may especially give patients with intrasellar tumors caused by prolactinoma at the pituitary gland. Transsphenoidal surgery subsides the reverse clinical symptoms, reduce high prolactin level, and normalize tumor size in patients with pituitary prolactinoma [95].

In addition, about 70 prolactinaemic patients with pituitary prolactinoma were diagnosed, but the success rate of the surgery depends upon the diameter, size of the adenoma, and prolactin level in blood serum. However, assessment of these two parameters may give a comprehensive conclusion as well as the prediction of endocrine results [96]. Another study exhibited that around 184 causes of male prolactinoma were examined and the following parameters were observed such as hormone levels, imaging features, clinical manifestations (dysfunction, headache, and visual disturbance), pathology results, preoperative treatments, surgical outcomes, *etc.* Bromocriptine sensitivity tests were conducted for all patients. Finding of the study (decreased prolactin level and increased dopamine level)indicate that in male prolactinoma patients, pituitary diameter and increased prolactin levels were reduced significantly [97]. Considering the facts, there are limited surgical tools available to subside the prolactinoma associated with hyperprolactinemia. Hence, there is a need to develop more precise surgical gears and other alternatives to overcome the adverse events associated with the neuroleptic drug.

Shortcomings in the Management of Hyperprolactinemia

The treatment outcome desired in hyperprolactinemia is to reduce the prolactin level. There is also a need to reduce tumor mass and prevent further disease proliferation. Dopamine agonists play a chief role in the management of hyperprolactinemia. The drugs acting on the dopamine receptor (D_2) in the pituitary gland (lactotroph cells) leads to downregulating the release of prolactin level [98, 99]. Dopamine agonists including apomorphine, pergolide, ropinirole, bromocriptine, cabergoline,quinagolide *etc* are used as a first-line therapy with keen objective to reduce hyperprolactinemia [100].

In pregnancy and the hyperprolactinaemic woman, dopaminergic agonist therapy should be withdrawn to avoid any possible teratogenic risk. Bromocriptine has been found to be safer in pregnancy. However, cabergoline and quinagolide are still limited use due to their adverse effect profile [101 - 103]. Further, in case of hyperprolactinemia, women's are intolerant to dopamine agonist due to hormonal and pregnancy associated side effect rather oestrogen-replacement therapy may be given to prevent further osteoporosis [104]. There is a need of regular management of prolactin level who use oral contraceptives [105]. However, in most cases olanzapine may be given because of lesser side effect on prolactin secretion [106, 107].

Ideal Drug for Management of Hyperprolactinemic

Among the existing drugs bromocriptine is used to reduce the prolactin level in 80-90% of patient with hyperprolactinemia [108 - 110]. However, about 60% of patients develop severe adverse events which included abdominal pain, dyspepsia, dizziness, headache and postural hypotension which limits their use [111]. Various studies have been done which suggested that bromocriptine in long term use causes intolerance and resistance [112, 113]. Cabergoline is also a preferable choice to reduce the hyperprolactinemia because of its better tolerability than bromocriptine [114, 115]. Presently quinagolide is alternative drug because of its effectiveness and safe therapeutic potential.

Resistance is an abbreviated term related to treatment failure during the continuation of treatment. Nonetheless, resistance to the dopamine receptor results in the failure of the reduction of the prolactin level [116]. So, in this connection, a recent study revealed that nearly 20% hyperprolactinemic patients and 30% macroprolactinoma patients treated with bromocriptine failed to reduce the prolactin level whereas 10%-20% of patients treated with cabergoline were better in condition [117, 118]. Because of the limited therapeutic utility of dopamine agonists, there is a need to look forward to the alternate therapy to minimize the side effect of neuroleptic drugs. So, the medicinal plants such as *B. monosperma* and *T. cordifolia* may be a suitable alternative in the management of hyperprolactinemia.

CONCLUSION

Hyperprolactinemia is a major side effect associated with neuroleptic drugs used in the treatment of schizophrenia. Use of dopaminergic agonists for the treatment of neuroleptic drug-induced hyperprolactinemia may compromise the efficacy of neuroleptic drugs. So, there is a need to develop drugs for neuroleptic drug-induced hyperprolactinemia which should not affect dopaminergic function. Screening with animal models is the first step in the drug discovery process. Lack of suitable animal models for evaluation of neuroleptic drug-induced hyperprolactinemia may be one of the reasons for the non-availability of suitable drugs.

Available animal models use prolactin (5 mg/kg/day for 1 week), haloperidol (1, 2 & 5 mg/kg/day for 16 days), metoclopramide (24 mg/kg for five days, 75 mg/kg for 15 days, 150 mg/kg/day for 10 days and 50 mg/kg/day for 5 days) and sulpiride (20, 40 mg/kg/day for 28 days and 20, 40 mg/kg/day for 30 and 60 days). These animal models are associated with ambiguity with respect to the dose of chemicals, sex of animals, *etc.* So, we suggest that there is a need to develop new models or validate available preclinical models to counter the neuroleptic drug-induced hyperprolactinemia. These animal models may also encourage research on other complications associated with antipsychotic drugs.

ABBREVIATIONS

(EPS)   Extrapyramidal side effects

(MAPK) Mitogen-activated protein kinase

(PRL)   Prolactin

(FSH)	Follicle-stimulating hormone
(LH)	Luteinizing hormone
(HPL)	Haloperidol
(MCP)	Metoclopramide

CONSENT FOR PUBLICATION

Not applicable.

CONFLICT OF INTEREST

The authors confirm that the contents of this chapter have no conflict of interest.

ACKNOWLEDGEMENTS

The authors wish to thank Indian Council of Medical Research (ICMR), New Delhi, India (45/5/2013/BMS/TRM) for providing financial assistantship in the form of fellowship and Regional Medical Research Center (RMRC), Bhubaneswar for providing library facilities.

REFERENCES

[1]   Di Luca M, Nutt D, Oertel W, *et al.* Towards earlier diagnosis and treatment of disorders of the brain. Bull World Health Organ 2018; 96(5): 298-298A.
[http://dx.doi.org/10.2471/BLT.17.206599] [PMID: 29875510]

[2]   Perry DC, Sturm VE, Peterson MJ, *et al.* Association of traumatic brain injury with subsequent neurological and psychiatric disease: a meta-analysis. J Neurosurg 2016; 124(2): 511-26.
[http://dx.doi.org/10.3171/2015.2.JNS14503] [PMID: 26315003]

[3]   Buckley PF, Miller BJ, Lehrer DS, Castle DJ. Psychiatric comorbidities and schizophrenia. Schizophr Bull 2009; 35(2): 383-402.
[http://dx.doi.org/10.1093/schbul/sbn135] [PMID: 19011234]

[4]   Mitchell AJ, Selmes T. Why don't patients attend their appointments? Maintaining engagement with psychiatric services. Adv Psychiatr Treat 2007; 13(6): 423-34.
[http://dx.doi.org/10.1192/apt.bp.106.003202]

[5]   Crismon L, Argo TR, Buckley PF. Schizophrenia.Pharmacotherapy: A Pathophysiologic Approach. 9th ed. New York, New York: McGraw-Hill 2014; pp. 1019-46.

[6]   Beck A, Rector N, Stolar N, *et al.* Schizophrenia: Cognitive theory, research, and therapy. Psychiatr Rehabil J 2009; 32: 327-8.
[http://dx.doi.org/10.1037/h0094638]

[7]   Lavretsky H. History of Schizophrenia as a Psychiatric Disorder.Clinical Handbook of Schizophrenia. History of Schizophrenia as a Psychiatric Disorder. In: Mueser KT, Jeste DVClinical Handbook of Schizophrenia. New York, New York: Guilford Press 2008; pp. 3-12.

[8]   Wu EQ, Shi L, Birnbaum H, Hudson T, Kessler R. Annual prevalence of diagnosed schizophrenia in the USA: a claims data analysis approach. Psychol Med 2006; 36(11): 1535-40.
[http://dx.doi.org/10.1017/S0033291706008191] [PMID: 16907994]

[9]   Finkel T, Deng CX, Mostoslavsky R. Recent progress in the biology and physiology of sirtuins.

Nature 2009; 460(7255): 587-91.
[http://dx.doi.org/10.1038/nature08197] [PMID: 19641587]

[10]   Volavka J, Czobor P, Sheitman B. risperidone, and haloperidol in the treatment of patients with chronic schizophrenia and schizoaffective disorder Am J Psychiatry1 2002; 159: 255-62.

[11]   King C, Voruganti LN. What's in a name? The evolution of the nomenclature of antipsychotic drugs. J Psychiatry Neurosci 2002; 27(3): 168-75.
[PMID: 12066446]

[12]   Smith FA, Wittmann CW, Stern TA. Medical complications of psychiatric treatment. Crit Care Clin 2008; 24(4): 635-656, vii.
[http://dx.doi.org/10.1016/j.ccc.2008.05.004] [PMID: 18929938]

[13]   Umbricht D, Kane JM. Medical complications of new antipsychotic drugs. Schizophr Bull 1996; 22(3): 475-83.
[http://dx.doi.org/10.1093/schbul/22.3.475] [PMID: 8873298]

[14]   Wagstaff A, Perry C. Clozapine: in prevention of suicide in patients with schizophrenia or schizoaffective disorder. CNS Drugs 2003; 17(4): 273-80.
[http://dx.doi.org/10.2165/00023210-200317040-00004] [PMID: 12665398]

[15]   Molitch ME. Medication-induced hyperprolactinemia. Mayo Clin Proc 2005; 80(8): 1050-7.
[http://dx.doi.org/10.4065/80.8.1050] [PMID: 16092584]

[16]   Haddad PM, Wieck A. Antipsychotic-induced hyperprolactinemia. Drugs 2004; 64: 2291-314.
[http://dx.doi.org/10.2165/00003495-200464200-00003] [PMID: 15456328]

[17]   Inder WJ, Castle D. Antipsychotic-induced hyperprolactinaemia. Aust N Z J Psychiatry 2011; 45(10): 830-7.
[http://dx.doi.org/10.3109/00048674.2011.589044] [PMID: 21714721]

[18]   Freeman ME, Kanyicska B, Lerant A, Nagy G. Prolactin: structure, function, and regulation of secretion. Physiol Rev 2000; 80(4): 1523-631.
[http://dx.doi.org/10.1152/physrev.2000.80.4.1523] [PMID: 11015620]

[19]   Flint DJ, Binart N, Kopchick J, Kelly P. Effects of growth hormone and prolactin on adipose tissue development and function. Pituitary 2003; 6(2): 97-102.
[http://dx.doi.org/10.1023/B:PITU.0000004800.57449.67] [PMID: 14703019]

[20]   Nilsson LA, Roepstorff C, Kiens B, Billig H, Ling C. Prolactin suppresses malonyl-CoA concentration in human adipose tissue. Horm Metab Res 2009; 41(10): 747-51.
[http://dx.doi.org/10.1055/s-0029-1224181] [PMID: 19551610]

[21]   Findling RL, Kusumakar V, Daneman D, Moshang T, De Smedt G, Binder C. Prolactin levels during long-term risperidone treatment in children and adolescents. J Clin Psychiatry 2003; 64(11): 1362-9.
[http://dx.doi.org/10.4088/JCP.v64n1113] [PMID: 14658952]

[22]   Dorshkind K, Horseman ND. Anterior pituitary hormones, stress, and immune system homeostasis. Bioessays 200 23(3): 94-4.
[http://dx.doi.org/10.1002/1521-1878(200103)23:3<288::AID-BIES1039>3.0.CO;2-P]

[23]   Gorvin CM. The prolactin receptor: Diverse and emerging roles in pathophysiology. J Clin Transl Endocrinol 2015; 2(3): 85-91.
[http://dx.doi.org/10.1016/j.jcte.2015.05.001] [PMID: 29204371]

[24]   Philips N, McFadden K. Inhibition of transforming growth factor-beta and matrix metalloproteinases by estrogen and prolactin in breast cancer cells. Cancer Lett 2004; 206(1): 63-8.
[http://dx.doi.org/10.1016/j.canlet.2003.10.019] [PMID: 15019161]

[25]   Harris J, Stanford PM, Oakes SR, Ormandy CJ. Prolactin and the prolactin receptor: new targets of an old hormone. Ann Med 2004; 36(6): 414-25.
[http://dx.doi.org/10.1080/07853890410033892] [PMID: 15513293]

[26]   Mancini T, Casanueva FF, Giustina A. Hyperprolactinemia and prolactinomas. Endocrinol Metab Clin North Am 2008; 37(1): 67-99, viii.
[http://dx.doi.org/10.1016/j.ecl.2007.10.013] [PMID: 18226731]

[27]   Utama FE, LeBaron MJ, Neilson LM, *et al.* Human prolactin receptors are insensitive to mouse prolactin: implications for xenotransplant modeling of human breast cancer in mice. J Endocrinol 2006; 188(3): 589-601.
[http://dx.doi.org/10.1677/joe.1.06560] [PMID: 16522738]

[28]   Macias H, Hinck L. Mammary gland development. Wiley Interdiscip Rev Dev Biol 2012; 1(4): 533-57.
[http://dx.doi.org/10.1002/wdev.35] [PMID: 22844349]

[29]   Melkersson K. Differences in prolactin elevation and related symptoms of atypical antipsychotics in schizophrenic patients. J Clin Psychiatry 2005; 66(6): 761-7.
[http://dx.doi.org/10.4088/JCP.v66n0614] [PMID: 15960571]

[30]   Yun BY, Cho C, Cho BN. Differential activity of 16K rat prolactin in different organic systems. Anim Cells Syst (Seoul) 2019; 23(2): 135-42.
[http://dx.doi.org/10.1080/19768354.2018.1554543] [PMID: 30949401]

[31]   Bardoloi PS. Review of Treatment option of Psychiatric Symptoms in a Case of functional Neuroendocrine Tumor. J Neurooncol Neurscience 2018; 3(1): 1.

[32]   Casanueva FF, Molitch ME, Schlechte JA, *et al.* Guidelines of the Pituitary Society for the diagnosis and management of prolactinomas. Clini endocrinol 2006; 65: 265-723.

[33]   Serri O, Chik CL, Ur E, Ezzat S. Diagnosis and management of hyperprolactinemia. CMAJ 2003; 169(6): 575-81.
[PMID: 12975226]

[34]   Isah I, Aliyu I, Yusuf R, *et al.* Hyperprolactinemia and female infertility: Pattern of clinical presentation in a tertiary health facility in Northern Nigeria. Sahel Med J 2018; 21: 1.
[http://dx.doi.org/10.4103/smj.smj_69_15]

[35]   Wattegama MH, Siyambalapitiya S. Drug induced hyperprolactinemia. Sri Lanka J Diabetes Endocrinol Metab 2017; 7: 26-32.
[http://dx.doi.org/10.4038/sjdem.v7i2.7333]

[36]   Bostwick JR, Guthrie SK, Ellingrod VL. Antipsychotic□induced hyperprolactinemia. Pharmacotherapy: *The J Human Pharmacol.* Drug Ther 2009; 29: 64-73.

[37]   Ajmal A, Joffe H, Nachtigall LB. Psychotropic-induced hyperprolactinemia: a clinical review. Psychosomatics 2014; 55(1): 29-36.
[http://dx.doi.org/10.1016/j.psym.2013.08.008] [PMID: 24140188]

[38]   Lippi G, Plebani M. Macroprolactin: searching for a needle in a haystack? Clin Chem Lab Med 2016; 54(4): 519-22.
[http://dx.doi.org/10.1515/cclm-2015-1283] [PMID: 26845727]

[39]   Torre DL, Falorni A. Pharmacological causes of hyperprolactinemia. Ther Clin Risk Manag 2007; 3(5): 929-51.
[PMID: 18473017]

[40]   Woitowich NC, Philibert KD, Leitermann RJ, Wungjiranirun M, Urban JH, Glucksman MJ. EP24. 15 as a potential regulator of kisspeptin within the neuroendocrine hypothalamus. Endocrinology 2016; 157(2): 820-30.
[http://dx.doi.org/10.1210/en.2015-1580] [PMID: 26653570]

[41]   Mateos J, Mañanos E, Carrillo M, Zanuy S. Regulation of follicle-stimulating hormone (FSH) and luteinizing hormone (LH) gene expression by gonadotropin-releasing hormone (GnRH) and sexual steroids in the Mediterranean Sea bass. Comp Biochem Physiol B Biochem Mol Biol 2002; 132(1):

75-86.
[http://dx.doi.org/10.1016/S1096-4959(01)00535-8] [PMID: 11997211]

[42]   Cohen LG, Biederman J. Treatment of risperidone-induced hyperprolactinemia with a dopamine agonist in children. J Child Adolesc Psychopharmacol 2001; 11(4): 435-40.
[http://dx.doi.org/10.1089/104454601317261618] [PMID: 11838826]

[43]   Perkins DO. Antipsychotic-induced hyperprolactinemia: pathophysiology and clinical consequences. Adv Stud Med 2004; 4(10F): S982-6.

[44]   Chahal J, Schlechte J. Hyperprolactinemia. Pituitary 2008; 11(2): 141-6.
[http://dx.doi.org/10.1007/s11102-008-0107-5] [PMID: 18404389]

[45]   Besnard I, Auclair V, Callery G, Gabriel-Bordenave C, Roberge C. [Antipsychotic-drug-induced hyperprolactinemia: physiopathology, clinical features and guidance]. Encephale 2014; 40(1): 86-94.
[http://dx.doi.org/10.1016/j.encep.2012.03.002] [PMID: 23928066]

[46]   Halbreich U, Kahn LS. Hormonal aspects of schizophrenias: an overview. Psychoneuroendocrinology 2003; 28 (Suppl. 2): 1-16.
[PMID: 12650679]

[47]   Gómez F, Reyes FI, Faiman C. Nonpuerperal galactorrhea and hyperprolactinemia. Clinical findings, endocrine features and therapeutic responses in 56 cases. Am J Med 1977; 62(5): 648-60.
[PMID: 558726]

[48]   Zhao J, Song X, Ai X, *et al.* Adjunctive aripiprazole treatment for risperidone-induced hyperprolactinemia: an 8-week randomized, open-label, comparative clinical trial. PLoS One 2015; 10(10)e0139717
[http://dx.doi.org/10.1371/journal.pone.0139717] [PMID: 26448615]

[49]   Anderson GM, Scahill L, McCracken JT, *et al.* Effects of short- and long-term risperidone treatment on prolactin levels in children with autism. Biol Psychiatry 2007; 61(4): 545-50.
[http://dx.doi.org/10.1016/j.biopsych.2006.02.032] [PMID: 16730335]

[50]   Kearns AE, Goff DC, Hayden DL, Daniels GH. Risperidone-associated hyperprolactinemia. Endocr Pract 2000; 6(6): 425-9.
[http://dx.doi.org/10.4158/EP.6.6.425] [PMID: 11155212]

[51]   Paparrigopoulos T, Liappas J, Tzavellas E, Mourikis I, Soldatos C. Amisulpride-induced hyperprolactinemia is reversible following discontinuation. Prog Neuropsychopharmacol Biol Psychiatry 2007; 31(1): 92-6.
[http://dx.doi.org/10.1016/j.pnpbp.2006.07.006] [PMID: 16938372]

[52]   Lee BH, Kang SG, Kim TW, Lee HJ, Yoon HK, Park YM. Hyperprolactinemia induced by low-dosage amisulpride in Korean psychiatric patients. Psychiatry Clin Neurosci 2012; 66(1): 69-73.
[http://dx.doi.org/10.1111/j.1440-1819.2011.02296.x] [PMID: 22250612]

[53]   Kuchay MS, Mithal A. Levosulpiride and serum prolactin levels. Indian J Endocrinol Metab 2017; 21(2): 355-8.
[http://dx.doi.org/10.4103/ijem.IJEM_555_16] [PMID: 28459037]

[54]   David SR, Taylor CC, Kinon BJ, Breier A. The effects of olanzapine, risperidone, and haloperidol on plasma prolactin levels in patients with schizophrenia. Clin Ther 2000; 22(9): 1085-96.
[http://dx.doi.org/10.1016/S0149-2918(00)80086-7] [PMID: 11048906]

[55]   Wang D, Wong HK, Zhang L, *et al.* Not only dopamine D2 receptors involved in Peony-Glycyrrhiza Decoction, an herbal preparation against antipsychotic-associated hyperprolactinemia. Prog Neuropsychopharmacol Biol Psychiatry 2012; 39(2): 332-8.
[http://dx.doi.org/10.1016/j.pnpbp.2012.07.005] [PMID: 22796279]

[56]   Biller BM, Luciano A, Crosignani PG, *et al.* Guidelines for the diagnosis and treatment of hyperprolactinemia. J Reprod Med 1999; 44(12) (Suppl.): 1075-84.
[PMID: 10649814]

[57] Colao A, Di Sarno A, Guerra E, De Leo M, Mentone A, Lombardi G. Drug insight: Cabergoline and bromocriptine in the treatment of hyperprolactinemia in men and women. Nat Clin Pract Endocrinol Metab 2006; 2(4): 200-10.
[http://dx.doi.org/10.1038/ncpendmet0160] [PMID: 16932285]

[58] Tollin SR. Use of the dopamine agonists bromocriptine and cabergoline in the management of risperidone-induced hyperprolactinemia in patients with psychotic disorders. J Endocrinol Invest 2000; 23(11): 765-70.
[http://dx.doi.org/10.1007/BF03345068] [PMID: 11194712]

[59] Lobo RA, Kletzky OA. Normalization of androgen and sex hormone-binding globulin levels after treatment of hyperprolactinemia. J Clin Endocrinol Metab 1983; 56(3): 562-6.
[http://dx.doi.org/10.1210/jcem-56-3-562] [PMID: 6296189]

[60] Schade R, Andersohn F, Suissa S, Haverkamp W, Garbe E. Dopamine agonists and the risk of cardiac-valve regurgitation. N Engl J Med 2007; 356(1): 29-38.
[http://dx.doi.org/10.1056/NEJMoa062222] [PMID: 17202453]

[61] Zanettini R, Antonini A, Gatto G, Gentile R, Tesei S, Pezzoli G. Valvular heart disease and the use of dopamine agonists for Parkinson's disease. N Engl J Med 2007; 356(1): 39-46.
[http://dx.doi.org/10.1056/NEJMoa054830] [PMID: 17202454]

[62] Darwish AM, Hafez E, El-Gebali I, Hassan SB, Ali ME. Rectal *versus* vaginal bromocriptine mesylate suppositories in hyperprolactinemic patients: an active comparator trial. Middle East Fertil Soc J 2007; 12(2): 104.

[63] Busso C, Fernández-Sánchez M, García-Velasco JA, *et al.* The non-ergot derived dopamine agonist quinagolide in prevention of early ovarian hyperstimulation syndrome in IVF patients: a randomized, double-blind, placebo-controlled trial. Hum Reprod 2010; 25(4): 995-1004.
[http://dx.doi.org/10.1093/humrep/deq005] [PMID: 20139430]

[64] Di Sarno A, Landi ML, Marzullo P, *et al.* The effect of quinagolide and cabergoline, two selective dopamine receptor type 2 agonists, in the treatment of prolactinomas. Clin Endocrinol (Oxf) 2000; 53(1): 53-60.
[http://dx.doi.org/10.1046/j.1365-2265.2000.01016.x] [PMID: 10931080]

[65] Schultz PN, Ginsberg L, McCutcheon IE, Samaan N, Leavens M, Gagel RF. Quinagolide in the management of prolactinoma. Pituitary 2000; 3(4): 239-49.
[http://dx.doi.org/10.1023/A:1012884214668] [PMID: 11788012]

[66] Colao A, di Sarno A, Pivonello R, di Somma C, Lombardi G. Dopamine receptor agonists for treating prolactinomas. Expert Opin Investig Drugs 2002; 11(6): 787-800.
[http://dx.doi.org/10.1517/13543784.11.6.787] [PMID: 12036422]

[67] Leong KS, Foy PM, Swift AC, *et al.* CSF rhinorrhoea following treatment with dopamine agonists for massive invasive prolactinomas. *Clin endocrinolo*2000; 52: 43-49. Meisenzahl EM, Schmitt GJ, Scheuerecker J, Möller HJ. The role of dopamine for the pathophysiology of schizophrenia. Int Rev Psychiatry 2007; 19(4): 337-45.
[PMID: 17671867]

[68] Lieberman JA. Dopamine partial agonists: a new class of antipsychotic. CNS Drugs 2004; 18(4): 251-67.
[http://dx.doi.org/10.2165/00023210-200418040-00005] [PMID: 15015905]

[69] Rehman J, Christ G, Alyskewycz M, Kerr E, Melman A. Experimental hyperprolactinemia in a rat model: alteration in centrally mediated neuroerectile mechanisms. Int J Impot Res 2000; 12(1): 23-32.
[http://dx.doi.org/10.1038/sj.ijir.3900473] [PMID: 10982309]

[70] Kumar SK, Abhishek P, Kumar SP, *et al.* Study of oestrus cycle periodicity and oogenesis of adult albino rats: Response to hyperprolactinemia induced by haloperidol. Asian Pac J Reprod 2013; 2: 99-104.

[http://dx.doi.org/10.1016/S2305-0500(13)60127-X]

[71]   Thorat VM, Khanwelkar CC, Matule SM, *et al.* Effect of Mirtazapine Pre-treatment on Haloperidol, Ergometrine and Fluoxetine Induced Behaviours in Albino Rats. J Krishna Inst Med Sci 2019; 8: 61-72.

[72]   Tiwari P, Dubey SK, Sahu PK. *Butea monosperma* Reduces Haloperidol and Sulpiride Induced Hyperprolactinemia in Rats. J Krishna Inst Med Sci 2019; 8: 40-52.

[73]   Tiwari P, Dubey SK, Sahu PK. *Tinospora cordifolia* attenuates antipsychotic drug induced Hyperprolactinemia. Asian Pac J Reprod 2019; 8: 116-24.
[http://dx.doi.org/10.4103/2305-0500.259171]

[74]   Ye Q, Zhang QY, Zheng CJ, Wang Y, Qin LP. Casticin, a flavonoid isolated from Vitex rotundifolia, inhibits prolactin release *in vivo* and *in vitro*. Acta Pharmacol Sin 2010; 31(12): 1564-8.
[http://dx.doi.org/10.1038/aps.2010.178] [PMID: 21042288]

[75]   Wang AT, Mullan RJ, Lane MA, *et al.* Treatment of hyperprolactinemia: a systematic review and meta-analysis. Syst Rev 2012; 1: 33.
[http://dx.doi.org/10.1186/2046-4053-1-33] [PMID: 22828169]

[76]   Wei Y, Wang X, Yu Z, *et al.* Efficacy and Mechanism of Action of Yiru Tiaojing Granule Against Hyperprolactinemia *in vitro* and *in vivo*. Planta Med 2015; 81(14): 1255-62.
[http://dx.doi.org/10.1055/s-0035-1546208] [PMID: 26252831]

[77]   Hu Y, Xin HL, Zhang QY, Zheng HC, Rahman K, Qin LP. Anti-nociceptive and anti-hyperprolactinemia activities of Fructus Viticis and its effective fractions and chemical constituents. Phytomedicine 2007; 14(10): 668-74.
[http://dx.doi.org/10.1016/j.phymed.2007.01.008] [PMID: 17350238]

[78]   Wang X, Chen YG, Ma L, *et al.* Effect of Chinese medical herbs-Huiru Yizeng Yihao on hyperprolactinemia and hyperplasia of mammary gland in mice. Afr J Tradit Complement Altern Med 2013; 10(4): 24-35.
[http://dx.doi.org/10.4314/ajtcam.v10i4.5] [PMID: 24146497]

[79]   Mostafapour S, Zare S, Sadrkhanlou RA, Ahmadi A, Razi M. Sulpiride-induced hyperprolactinemia in mature female rats: evidence for alterations in the reproductive system, pituitary and ovarian hormones. Int J Fertil Steril 2014; 8(2): 193-206.
[PMID: 25083185]

[80]   Van Coppenolle F, Slomianny C, Carpentier F, *et al.* Effects of hyperprolactinemia on rat prostate growth: evidence of androgeno-dependence. Am J Physiol Endocrinol Metab 2001; 280(1): E120-9.
[http://dx.doi.org/10.1152/ajpendo.2001.280.1.E120] [PMID: 11120666]

[81]   Devin JK, Lakhani VT, Byrd BF III, Blevins LS Jr. Prevalence of valvular heart disease in a cohort of patients taking cabergoline for management of hyperprolactinemia. Endocr Pract 2008; 14(6): 672-7.
[http://dx.doi.org/10.4158/EP.14.6.672] [PMID: 18996784]

[82]   Melmed S, Casanueva FF, Hoffman AR, *et al.* Endocrine Society. Diagnosis and treatment of hyperprolactinemia: an Endocrine Society clinical practice guideline. J Clin Endocrinol Metab 2011; 96(2): 273-88.
[http://dx.doi.org/10.1210/jc.2010-1692] [PMID: 21296991]

[83]   Biller BM, Molitch ME, Vance ML, *et al.* Treatment of prolactin-secreting macroadenomas with the once-weekly dopamine agonist cabergoline. J Clin Endocrinol Metab 1996; 81(6): 2338-43.
[PMID: 8964874]

[84]   Verhelst J, Abs R, Maiter D, *et al.* Cabergoline in the treatment of hyperprolactinemia: a study in 455 patients. J Clin Endocrinol Metab 1999; 84(7): 2518-22.
[http://dx.doi.org/10.1210/jcem.84.7.5810] [PMID: 10404830]

[85]   Thorner MO. Prolactin: Clinical physiology and the significance and management of hyperprolactinemia. Clinical neuroendocrinology 1977; 61-319.

[86]   Marken PA, Haykal RF, Fisher JN. Management of psychotropic-induced hyperprolactinemia. Clin Pharm 1992; 11(10): 851-6.
[PMID: 1341991]

[87]   Vance ML, Evans WS, Thorner MO. Drugs five years later. Bromocriptine. Ann Intern Med 1984; 100(1): 78-91.
[http://dx.doi.org/10.7326/0003-4819-100-1-78] [PMID: 6229205]

[88]   Vance ML, Lipper M, Klibanski A, Biller BM, Samaan NA, Molitch ME. Treatment of prolactin-secreting pituitary macroadenomas with the long-acting non-ergot dopamine agonist CV 205-502. Ann Intern Med 1990; 112(9): 668-73.
[http://dx.doi.org/10.7326/0003-4819-112-9-668] [PMID: 1970714]

[89]   Thorner MO. Prolactin: Clinical physiology and the significance and management of hyperprolactinemia. Clinical neuroendocrinology 1977; 1: 61-319.

[90]   Soto-Albors CE, Randolph JF, Ying YK, Riddick DH. Medical management of hyperprolactinemia: a lower dose of bromocriptine may be effective. Fertil Steril 1987; 48(2): 213-7.
[http://dx.doi.org/10.1016/S0015-0282(16)59344-3] [PMID: 3609332]

[91]   van der Lely AJ, Brownell J, Lamberts SW. The efficacy and tolerability of CV 205-502 (a nonergot dopaminergic drug) in macroprolactinoma patients and in prolactinoma patients intolerant to bromocriptine. J Clin Endocrinol Metab 1991; 72(5): 1136-41.
[http://dx.doi.org/10.1210/jcem-72-5-1136] [PMID: 1673685]

[92]   Leong KS, Foy PM, Swift AC, Atkin SL, Hadden DR, MacFarlane IA. CSF rhinorrhoea following treatment with dopamine agonists for massive invasive prolactinomas. Clin endocrinolo 2000; 52(1): 43-9.
[http://dx.doi.org/10.1046/j.1365-2265.2000.00901.x]

[93]   Davis JR, Sheppard MC, Heath DA. Giant invasive prolactinoma: a case report and review of nine further cases. Q J Med 1990; 74(275): 227-38.
[PMID: 2385731]

[94]   Vilar L, Abucham J, Albuquerque JL, *et al.* Controversial issues in the management of hyperprolactinemia and prolactinomas - An overview by the Neuroendocrinology Department of the Brazilian Society of Endocrinology and Metabolism. Arch Endocrinol Metab 2018; 62(2): 236-63.
[http://dx.doi.org/10.20945/2359-3997000000032] [PMID: 29768629]

[95]   Losa M, Mortini P, Barzaghi R, Gioia L, Giovanelli M. Surgical treatment of prolactin-secreting pituitary adenomas: early results and long-term outcome. J Clin Endocrinol Metab 2002; 87(7): 3180-6.
[http://dx.doi.org/10.1210/jcem.87.7.8645] [PMID: 12107221]

[96]   Landolt AM. Surgical treatment of pituitary prolactinomas: postoperative prolactin and fertility in seventy patients. Fertil Steril 1981; 35(6): 620-5.
[http://dx.doi.org/10.1016/S0015-0282(16)45552-4] [PMID: 7250389]

[97]   Song YJ, Chen MT, Lian W, *et al.* Surgical treatment for male prolactinoma: A retrospective study of 184 cases 2017.
[http://dx.doi.org/10.1097/MD.0000000000005833]

[98]   De Camilli P, Macconi D, Spada A. Dopamine inhibits adenylate cyclase in human prolactin-secreting pituitary adenomas. Nature 1979; 278(5701): 252-4.
[http://dx.doi.org/10.1038/278252a0] [PMID: 423973]

[99]   Vallar L, Vicentini LM, Meldolesi J. Inhibition of inositol phosphate production is a late, Ca2+-dependent effect of D2 dopaminergic receptor activation in rat lactotroph cells. J Biol Chem 1988; 263(21): 10127-34.
[PMID: 2839476]

[100]   Sachdev PS. The current status of tardive dyskinesia. Aust N Z J Psychiatry 2000; 34(3): 355-69.

[http://dx.doi.org/10.1080/j.1440-1614.2000.00737.x] [PMID: 10881961]

[101] Krupp P, Monka C. Bromocriptine in pregnancy: safety aspects. Klin Wochenschr 1987; 65(17): 823-7.
[http://dx.doi.org/10.1007/BF01727477] [PMID: 3657044]

[102] Raymond JP, Goldstein E, Konopka P, Leleu MF, Merceron RE, Loria Y. Follow-up of children born of bromocriptine-treated mothers. Horm Res 1985; 22(3): 239-46.
[http://dx.doi.org/10.1159/000180100] [PMID: 4054844]

[103] Molitch ME. Management of prolactinomas during pregnancy. J Reprod Med 1999; 44(12) (Suppl.): 1121-6.
[PMID: 10649822]

[104] Corenblum B, Donovan L. The safety of physiological estrogen plus progestin replacement therapy and with oral contraceptive therapy in women with pathological hyperprolactinemia. Fertil Steril 1993; 59(3): 671-3.
[http://dx.doi.org/10.1016/S0015-0282(16)55819-1] [PMID: 8458475]

[105] Garcia MM, Kapcala LP. Growth of a microprolactinoma to a macroprolactinoma during estrogen therapy. J Endocrinol Invest 1995; 18(6): 450-5.
[http://dx.doi.org/10.1007/BF03349744] [PMID: 7594240]

[106] Karagianis JL, Baksh A. High-dose olanzapine and prolactin levels. J Clin Psychiatry 2003; 64(10): 1192-4.
[http://dx.doi.org/10.4088/JCP.v64n1008] [PMID: 14658967]

[107] Wieck A, Haddad PM. Antipsychotic-induced hyperprolactinaemia in women: pathophysiology, severity and consequences. Selective literature review. Br J Psychiatry 2003; 182: 199-204.
[http://dx.doi.org/10.1192/bjp.182.3.199] [PMID: 12611781]

[108] Molitch ME, Elton RL, Blackwell RE, *et al.* Bromocriptine as primary therapy for prolactin-secreting macroadenomas: results of a prospective multicenter study. J Clin Endocrinol Metab 1985; 60(4): 698-705.
[http://dx.doi.org/10.1210/jcem-60-4-698] [PMID: 3882737]

[109] Vance ML, Evans WS, Thorner MO. Drugs five years later. Bromocriptine. Ann Intern Med 1984; 100(1): 78-91.
[http://dx.doi.org/10.7326/0003-4819-100-1-78] [PMID: 6229205]

[110] Bevan JS, Webster J, Burke CW, Scanlon MF. Dopamine agonists and pituitary tumor shrinkage. Endocr Rev 1992; 13(2): 220-40.
[http://dx.doi.org/10.1210/edrv-13-2-220] [PMID: 1352243]

[111] Ho KY, Thorner MO. Therapeutic applications of bromocriptine in endocrine and neurological diseases. Drugs 1988; 36(1): 67-82.
[http://dx.doi.org/10.2165/00003495-198836010-00005] [PMID: 3063495]

[112] Duranteau L, Chanson P, Lavoinne A, Horlait S, Lubetzki J, Kuhn JM. Effect of the new dopaminergic agonist CV 205-502 on plasma prolactin levels and tumour size in bromocriptine-resistant prolactinomas. Clin Endocrinol (Oxf) 1991; 34(1): 25-9.
[http://dx.doi.org/10.1111/j.1365-2265.1991.tb01731.x] [PMID: 1672268]

[113] Wand GS. Diagnosis and management of hyperprolactinemia. Endocrinologist 2003; 13(1): 52-7.
[http://dx.doi.org/10.1097/00019616-200301000-00010]

[114] Delgrange E, Maiter D, Donckier J. Effects of the dopamine agonist cabergoline in patients with prolactinoma intolerant or resistant to bromocriptine

[115] Di Sarno A, Landi ML, Cappabianca P, *et al.* Resistance to cabergoline as compared with bromocriptine in hyperprolactinemia: prevalence, clinical definition, and therapeutic strategy. J Clin Endocrinol Metab 2001; 86(11): 5256-61.
[http://dx.doi.org/10.1210/jcem.86.11.8054] [PMID: 11701688]

[116]   Pellegrini I, Rasolonjanahary R, Gunz G, *et al.* Resistance to bromocriptine in prolactinomas. J Clin Endocrinol Metab 1989; 69(3): 500-9.
[http://dx.doi.org/10.1210/jcem-69-3-500] [PMID: 2760167]

[117]   Olafsdottir A, Schlechte J. Management of resistant prolactinomas. Nat Clin Pract Endocrinol Metab 2006; 2(10): 552-61.
[http://dx.doi.org/10.1038/ncpendmet0290] [PMID: 17024154]

[118]   Delgrange E, Trouillas J, Maiter D, Donckier J, Tourniaire J. Sex-related difference in the growth of prolactinomas: a clinical and proliferation marker study. J Clin Endocrinol Metab 1997; 82(7): 2102-7.
[http://dx.doi.org/10.1210/jc.82.7.2102] [PMID: 9215279]

CHAPTER 5

Glioma Imaging and Novel Agents

Mine Silindir-Gunay[*]

Hacettepe University, Faculty of Pharmacy, Department of Radiopharmacy, 06100, Sıhhiye, Ankara, Turkey

Abstract: Glioma is one of the most frequently observed and aggressive brain tumors. Glioma forms 50-60% of brain tumors including astrocytoma, oligodendroglioma, and glioblastoma. Although the integrity of the blood-brain barrier (BBB) is destroyed somehow in glioblastoma (high-grade glioma) patients, similar to many central nervous system diseases, the main anatomical obstacle remains BBB in effective diagnosis, imaging, and therapy.

The survival rate of glioblastoma patients is very low. Early and accurate diagnosis of glioma is essential for therapy chance. When compared with other techniques, non-invasive medical imaging methods provide high specificity and sensitivity. Although MRI is one of the most commonly used modalities in glioma diagnosis and imaging, it possesses limited differentiation in tumor recurrence and pseudoprogression after radiotherapy and combined chemotherapy. Improved MRI techniques can exhibit higher potential in evaluating the pathological features and grading of gliomas before treatment. As a novel method, molecular imaging techniques such as PET/CT can detect genetic mechanisms and related molecular and metabolic differentiation for accurate diagnosis of diseases.

^{18}F-FDG, one of the most commonly used PET radiopharmaceuticals, is highly accumulated in the cerebral cortex. Therefore, ^{18}F-FDG is a non-specific agent in glioma diagnosis and imaging. Non-specific radiopharmaceuticals are not sufficient depending on low sensitivity and specificity in early diagnosis and imaging of proliferation index of tumor cells, the place of hypoxic focuses, tumor load, differentiation of tumor/necrosis, and tumor/inflammation and therapy monitoring of glioma. Therefore, target-specific radiocontrast/contrast agents have been searched for accurate diagnosis, imaging, and therapy monitoring of glioma. Specific PET agents provide differentiation of tumor, necrosis, or inflammation. More specific glioma imaging agents including novel specific Gd or SPIO comprising MRI contrast agents, amino acid tracers like ^{18}F-FET, and peptide tracers like αvβ3 integrin specific ^{68}Ga-RGD and radiolabeled, targeted drug delivery systems have been searched for accurate and early diagnosis of all stages of glioma.

[*] **Corresponding author Mine Silindir-Gunay**: Hacettepe University, Faculty of Pharmacy, Department of Radiopharmacy, 06100, Sıhhiye, Ankara, Turkey; Tel: 00903123052152, Fax: 00903123114777; E-mail: mines@hacettepe.edu.tr

Keywords: Blood-brain barrier, Diagnosis, Enhanced-permeability and retention effect, Glioma, Glioma targeting, Imaging, Multifunctional drug delivery systems, Nanocarriers, Radiopharmaceuticals, Specific probes, Theranostics for glioma.

INTRODUCTION

Glioblastoma is one of the most commonly observed and aggressive brain tumors. It takes its roots from star-shaped glial tissues. Glial cells support nerves, protect the BBB and, ensure continuity. Glioma is an umbrella term comprising astrocytoma, oligodendroglioma, and glioblastoma. Glioma is originated from glial tissues which are called astrocytes that gained abnormal features and shapes [1 - 7].

Glioblastoma is the primary malignant brain tumor and has the worst therapy potential. World Health Organization (WHO) defines glioblastoma as the highest grade (IV grade) brain tumor [8]. Grading of diffuse glioma according to WHO 2007 was defined as Astrocytoma (Grade II), Oligodendroglioma (Grade II), Oligoastrocytoma (Grade II), Anaplastic-astrocytoma/oligodendroglioma (Grade III) and Glioblastoma (Grade IV) [8]. However, according to WHO 2016, molecular parameters in addition to histology have been initiated to use for the classification of CNS tumors. In this version, a major restructuring of the diffuse gliomas, medulloblastomas and other embryonal tumors was defined incorporating new entities based on both histology and molecular features such as glioblastoma, IDH-wildtype, and glioblastoma, IDH-mutant; diffuse midline glioma, H3 K27M–mutant; RELA fusion-positive ependymoma; medulloblastoma, WNT-activated and medulloblastoma, SHH-activated; and embryonal tumor with multilayered rosettes, C19MC-altered [9]. The incidence rate of glioma is 3.19 per 100,000 persons in the USA and a median age of 64 years. It is 1.6 times higher in males compared to females and it is uncommon in children [10].

This tumor may also attack both hemispheres of the brain [1 - 3]. It may also develop high vascularization into the surrounding brain parenchyma and extensive infiltration [4 - 7]. Therefore, survival is fairly poor for glioma patients. Only a few of them survive for 2.5 years following diagnosis [10]. However, early diagnosis and imaging of the disease are essential to enhance therapy efficacy and chances of survival. When compared with other techniques, non-invasive molecular imaging and advanced Magnetic Resonance Imaging (MRI) techniques possess high importance for the diagnosis of neurological diseases and alterations formed before and after tumor depending on high specificity and sensitivity. Molecular imaging provides information about monitoring of quantification of gene and protein functions, protein-protein interactions and signal transduction pathways, non-invasive detection, imaging and characterization related to the molecular pathophysiology of a specific disease [11, 12]. In this way, a more accurate and specific diagnosis of glioma can be obtained by the multidisciplinary cooperation of different branches including Nuclear Medicine, Radiology, Neurology, Neurosurgery, Oncology, and Pharmacy. To perform effective and specific molecular imaging, it is essential to establish molecular imaging probes conjugated with mAbs, antibody fragments, ligands, enzymes, substrates, peptides, proteins and markers that are specific to a receptor, amino acid or enzyme expressed in the target organ/tissue within the body. These probes can be used for imaging of the last product in the gene expression of a specific protein for binding to a target protein or markers after the radiolabeling process. These interactions are performed due to receptor-radionuclide binding or enzyme-radionuclide substrate reaction [12 - 14]. Recently, the design of novel radiocontrast/contrast agents for sensitive and accurate imaging is getting popular and attractive. Molecular imaging can detect *in vivo* mechanisms and cellular and molecular pathways of the diseases in a dynamic and reproducible way physiologically and directly [11].

MRI, having a high spatial resolution, is an essential imaging modality in the diagnosis and therapy monitoring of high-grade gliomas having high contrast. However, it is not a tumor-specific imaging method. The diagnostic criteria in glioma imaging of routinely used MRI depend on the contrast agent enhancement related to the disruption of the blood-brain barrier (BBB) penetration [15]. This disruption in BBB is generally formed after surgery or radiotherapy. However, BBB may remain intact in some tumor areas. Contrast enhancement can be observed lesser than the real tumor size especially at low-grade gliomas which may cause insufficient assessment. Additionally, novel therapeutic approaches such as vascular endothelial growth factor (VEGF) inhibitors can reduce the disruption of BBB which causes reduction of contrast enhancement in MRI. This is defined as pseudoregression. This effect can be observed after the administration of corticosteroids reducing the relaxation of blood vessels [16, 17].

Computed Tomography (CT) is one of the oldest radiological imaging techniques. Cross-sectional anatomical images are obtained by using X-rays. Positive and negative contrast agents can be used for contrast enhancement of tissues and organs to obtain accurate images. When compared with MRI, CT gives less detailed soft tissue images. Although routinely used MRI and CT are the most frequently used techniques to obtain anatomical alterations in glioma imaging, they are very limited in the differentiation of tumor necrosis and inflammation from tumor after therapy. However, Positron Emission Tomography (PET) imaging with the use of specific radiotracers provides functional information related to sufficient differentiation of necrosis and inflammation from tumor. Nowadays, the genetic mechanisms related to the disease and the detection of related molecular and metabolic alterations are essential to evaluate the real widespread of the tumor, the existence and the type of receptor, and metabolic pathway by target-specific agents. Nowadays, the use of target-specific contrast/radiocontrast agents has a significant role in the diagnosis and/or therapy and therapy monitoring of tumor within the concept of personalized medicine or precision medicine.

PET is an essential functional imaging modality and its use in the diagnosis and therapy monitoring of gliomas has achieved widespread utilization. Hybrid imaging modalities including PET/CT, SPECT/CT, PET/MRI combine anatomical and functional information on the images. In this way, the limitations of single modalities can be removed.

Although contrast and radiocontrast agents were given in detail in the related parts below, some specifically used PET tracers for glioma imaging were given briefly in this part. ^{18}F-FDG is one of the most commonly used PET radiopharmaceuticals for the diagnosis of several diseases. Due to a severe increase in glycolysis, ^{18}F-FDG is accumulated in high concentration giving high accumulation foci. However, ^{18}F-FDG is accumulated in high content in the cerebral cortex of the brain normally. The most important limitation of ^{18}F-FDG PET is that glucose is the normal substrate of the brain. Therefore, it causes a high false-negative result due to low lesion background contrast. In this way, ^{18}F-FDG is generally not a good option and a specific radiopharmaceutical for the diagnosis of glioma [18, 19].

Nowadays, radiolabeled amino acid tracers are one of the most commonly searched PET radiopharmaceuticals for imaging of brain tumors. The uptake of amino acids by normal brain tissue is rather low when compared with tumor tissue [20 - 22]. Amino acid uptake in the tumor tissue is mainly performed by type I-amino acid transporters [21]. It was reported that the transporter expression can especially be stimulated in the vasculature of brain tumors in the rat model [23]. Although [11C] Methionine ([11C]-MET) and [18]Fluoro-O-(2) fluoroethyl-l-tyrosine (^{18}F-FET) are the most commonly searched amino acid tracers for imaging of malignant brain tumors, their routine clinical applications stay still very limited when compared to ^{18}F-FDG [17].

It is widely known that tumor cells in enhanced proliferation state need more oxygen and new vascularization [24, 25]. Angiogenic alteration occurs with the release of several preangiogenic factors mainly vascular endothelial growth factor (VEGF) by endothelial, stromal, and tumor cells causing vascularization and tumor expansion [24]. High-grade glioma is one of the most vascularized human tumors [26].

Therefore, high-grade glioma cells produce proangiogenic factors including VEGF. VEGF is composed of 5 glycoprotein families, including VEGF-A, VEGF-B, VEGF-C, VEGF-D, and placental growth factors which are bound to the corresponding tyrosine kinase receptors (VEGFR-1, VEGFR-2, and VEGFR-3) and activate a flow signal causing angiogenesis, enhanced vascular permeability and lymphangiogenesis progress. VEGF-A plays the most important role in tumor angiogenesis. Enhanced levels of VEGF-A designate a bad prognosis in cancer patients [27, 28].

In the case of glioma treatment, chemotherapeutic agents, and monoclonal antibodies as single agents or as the combination can be used as significant alternatives. Bevacizumab is one of the most commonly used mAbs. It is a recombinant human-sourced monoclonal immunoglobulin G1 (IgG1) antibody against VEGF. It was taken an accelerated FDA approval in the USA as a single agent for the therapy of glioma recurrence. However, EMA refused this indication due to the lack of indication. While Bevacizumab is used as standard therapy for the treatment of glioma recurrence in the USA, it is not used in Europe. Bevacizumab is used as the primary treatment option and recurrence in phase II trials [29]. Recently, the results of phase III studies of Bevacizumab designated that the use of Bevacizumab in addition to standard radiotherapy and combination with adjuvant temozolomide therapy exhibited better prognosis in early diagnosed glioma patients. Besides, Bevacizumab enhances life quality in glioma patients. It selectively binds to all isoforms of human VEGF with a high affinity and neutralizes the biological activity of VEGF by blocking VEGF binding to VEGFR-1 and VEGFR-2 receptors on the surface of endothelial cells [29 - 31].

Temozolomide (TMZ) is standard of care for glioblastoma since 2005. It is also a standard of care of anaplastic astrocytoma and oligoastrocytoma in many places. TMZ is a new class of second-generation imidazaotetrazine prodrugs which spontaneously turns to active alkylating carboxymide (MTIC) at physiological conditions. Therefore, hepatic metabolism is not necessary for the activation of TMZ [32]. It was reported that TMZ designates antitumor activity in glioma, melanoma, and other high-grade tumors [33 - 35]. TMZ penetrates all tissues primarily the central nervous system (CNS) in preclinical studies [33 - 38].

BBB Obstacle and EPR Effect Advantage in Glioma Imaging and Therapy

BBB is the main obstacle in the diagnosis and/or therapy of gliomas like many brain tumors and neurological diseases. This barrier acts as a dynamic filter by preventing the penetration of many water-soluble drugs and also peptides, proteins, hormones to the CNS. Unlike endothelial cells in the peripheral tissues, tight junctions exist at BBB preventing solid and liquid transition freely [39, 40].

A schematic representation of the microenvironment of BBB is given in Fig. (**1**)

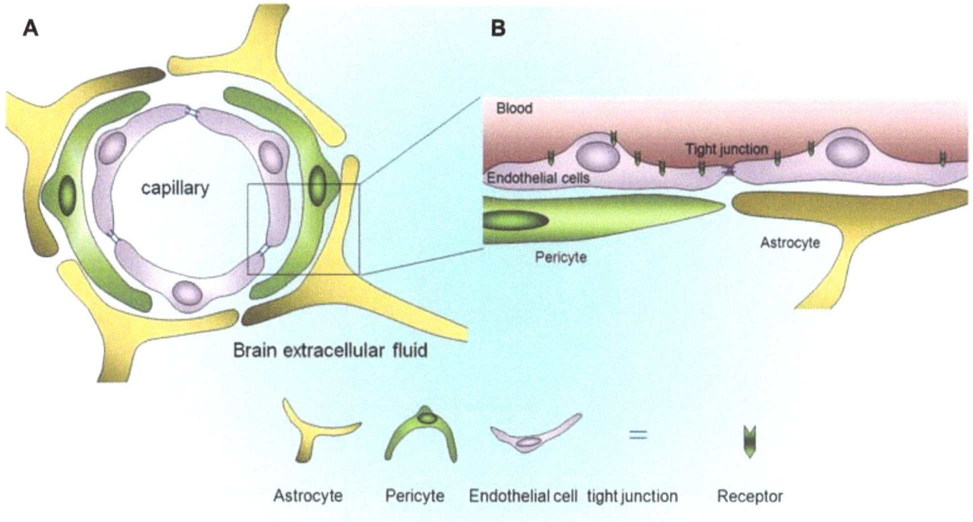

Fig. (1). Microenvironment of the BBB. (A) The diagram of the BBB *in vivo*. (B) Magnification of the BBB [41].

As it is widely known, BBB prevents the penetration of many pharmaceuticals having a large molecular weight and more than 98% of small molecular weight compounds as well. Targeted systems or agents have to be designed for BBB penetration to perform accurate diagnosis and/or therapy of many CNS diseases and tumors. The degree of BBB penetration depends on the lipophilicity, molecular weight, charge, and serum protein binding ratio of drugs or radiocontrast/contrast agents [42]. Radiocontrast/contrast agents that are used for CNS imaging have to possess some properties such as 1) ability to penetrate BBB (neutral, MW<700, log P:1-3), 2) *in vivo* stability, 3) ability to bind to the target receptor selectively, and 4) high accumulation in the brain.

Solid tumors generally have a diffusion-limited small size and remain at this size till angiogenesis. The process of neoangiogenesis provides the delivery of oxygen and nutrients to tumor cells for rapid proliferation [43]. Similar to tumors, this neovascularization is also leaky and lacks lymphatic drainage which provides several advantages to nanoparticle-based imaging probes and therapeutic agents for tumor targeting and accumulation [44 - 46]. This is known as the enhanced permeability and retention (EPR) effect [47]. EPR effect phenomenon does not comprise small molecular weight compounds as their uptake and distribution are performed by free diffusion. To benefit from the EPR effect, the particle size and surface properties of drug delivery systems have to be controlled for enhancing circulation time and preventing the reticuloendothelial system (RES) uptake. A schematic representation of probes benefited from the EPR effect is given in Fig. (**2**).

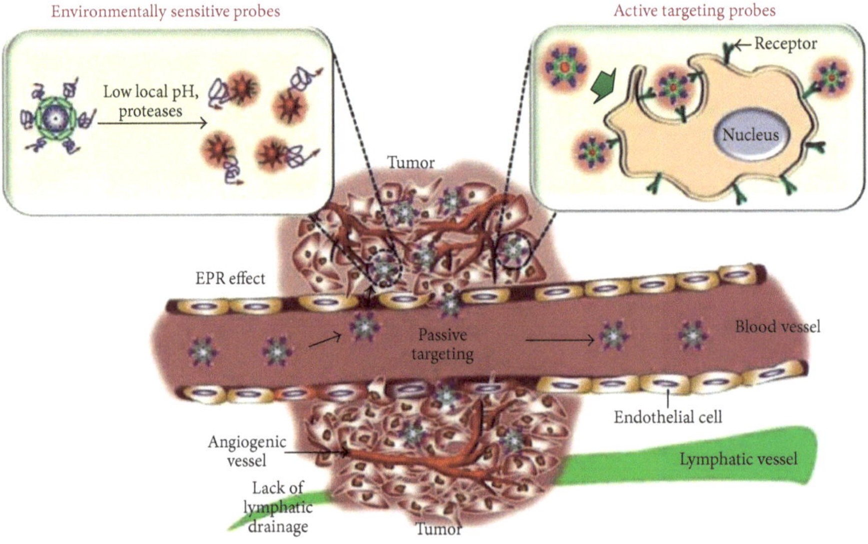

Fig. (2). The role of the EPR effect in tumor targeting of probes [48].

Glioma Imaging Modalities

As being one of the oldest modalities, CT is a radiological technique to obtain cross-sectional anatomical images by using X-rays. CT gives less detailed soft tissue images when compared with MRI. Positive and negative contrast agents are used for contrast enhancement to obtain accurate images. Positive contrast agents enhance tissue visualization by absorbing X-rays and give shiny images. These positive contrast agents generally include iodinated contrast agents such as iopromide, iohexol, iomeprole and, barium sulfate. Negative contrast agents such as air and CO_2 reduce tissue visualization. They penetrate X-rays and give dark images.

MRI is another anatomical imaging modality. It provides better soft tissue contrast than CT. Images of organs were obtained by the use of a strong magnetic field and radio waves. It is frequently used for the diagnosis and imaging of glioma in clinics. However, it is limited in the monitoring of therapy response and glioma recurrence. It is limited in the differentiation of pseudoprogression after radiotherapy and combined chemotherapy, especially in high-grade gliomas. Nowadays, diffusion, spectroscopy, perfusion MRI and functional MRI (fMRI) can provide images having more specific tissue characterization. Although these recent technologies possess a better and accurate diagnosis, they are not frequently used in routine clinic applications in many countries. MR images are obtained as T1-weighted and T2-weighted images according to T1 and T2 relaxation times that are the periods for returning of protons to the previous state after excitation with the radiowaves in 3D plane longitudinal and transverse directions, respectively. MRI contrast agents are classified as T1 agents and T2 agents. T1 agents include gadolinium such as gadobutrol, gadopentetate dimeglumin, gadodiamide, and gadoteric acid and mangan salts in which they provide bright images by reducing T1 relaxation times. T2 contrast agents include iron oxide agents such as superparamagnetic iron oxide nanoparticles (SPIONs) and ultra-small superparamagnetic iron oxide nanoparticles (USPIONs) having particle sizes higher than 50 nm and smaller than 50 nm, respectively. Therefore, while SPIONs can be used for RES imaging, USPIONs can be used for MR angiography, imaging of lymph nodes, and brain cancers. T2 contrast agents provide dark images by reducing T2 relaxation times. The use of contrast agents comprises a ratio of 25% among all routine investigations [49].

SPECT is a radionuclide mediated imaging technique. Upon the injection of a radiopharmaceutical having an appropriate gamma-emitting radionuclide, photons are accumulated in the collimators comprising position sensitive light detectors. Images were obtained after computer-aided processing. The use of collimators causes a significant reduction in detection efficiency. The spatial resolution and specificity of SPECT are lower than PET. $^{99m}TcO_4^-$, ^{99m}Tc-DTPA, ^{99m}Tc-HMPAO, ^{99m}Tc-ECD, ^{99m}Tc-Sestamibi, ^{99m}Tc-Tetraphosmine, ^{123}I-Alpha-Methyl-Tyrosine, ^{111}In-Pentetreotid, ^{201}Tl, ^{67}Ga-Citrate are radiopharmaceuticals that can be used for the detection of glioma due to enhanced metabolic activity and altered BBB penetration.

PET imaging is another radionuclide mediated molecular imaging technique providing imaging of cellular alterations before the formation of morphological alterations. PET images were obtained by the application of a positron-emitting radiopharmaceutical into the body. A photon couple is formed when the positron-emitting radionuclide interacts with the electrons of the atom. These photons having 511 keV energy move 180° angle opposite to each other. Afterward, these photons are captured by the detectors, and the image is formed after processing by a computer. The production of PET radionuclides generally needs more developed and expensive techniques when compared to SPECT radionuclides. However, higher resolution and sensitivity of the PET provide the detection of small lesions and artifacts. Additionally, functional and metabolic 3D images can be obtained. Glioma diagnosis, imaging, monitoring, determination of tumor expansion and border, biopsy planning, therapy planning, radiotherapy planning, and monitoring of therapy response can be performed by PET. Although PET provides many advantages, it is lack of anatomical information. Hybrid imaging modalities such as PET/CT and PET/MRI can overcome some of the disadvantages of PET such as lack of anatomical information [50]. By the fusion of anatomical and functional images, a more accurate diagnosis can be obtained. The use of these hybrid imaging modalities, patient comfort, and compliance can be enhanced by manipulating a single imaging protocol and reducing time. Therefore, it was observed that PET/CT and PET/MRI hybrid imaging modalities can be chosen as alternative applications to obtain a better resolution and anatomical correlation [51, 52]. Evaluation and imaging of glucose metabolism, amino acid transport, protein synthesis, proliferation rate, membrane biosynthesis, oxygen metabolism, and perfusion can be performed by PET for glioma imaging. Specifically targeted probes and ligands can be used for the evaluation of biological and biochemical processes after radiolabeling with PET radionuclides such as Carbon (^{11}C), Nitrogen (^{13}N), Oxygen (^{15}O) and Florine (^{18}F). When compared with PET radionuclides obtained from the cyclotron, ^{68}Ga is obtained from a ^{68}Ge-^{68}Ga generator easily for proper radiolabeling features and sufficient half-life (67.7 min.) [18]. The high positron emission fraction (89%, Emax: 1899 keV, Emean: 890 keV) and the proper half-life of ^{68}Ga provide high-quality images that make it a popular and a good option for PET imaging [19].

Glioma Imaging Agents

Molecular imaging is performed due to metabolic alterations within the body and frequently used for the diagnosis of brain tumors. Metabolism rate and expression of surface molecules and receptors of tumor cells are different than that of normal cells. Due to the differentiation grade, tumor cells lose their duty and synthesis functions. These cells stimulate protein and DNA synthesis for proliferation and also glycolysis to obtain the required energy which is in parallel with tumor malignancy. Some chemical biomolecules can be used for imaging of targeted metabolic pathways after radiolabeling. In this way, metabolic information can be obtained by the use of tumor sourced alterations [50].

Radioactive tracers or contrast agents used for molecular imaging are generally chosen from the molecules that are participated in the targeted pathways naturally. Radiocontrast agents are generally administered in tracer amounts which are different from other contrast agents used for other imaging modalities. These molecules are generally the substrates of the enzymes in targeted pathways or the ligands of targeted surface receptors [50]. Several contrast/radiocontrast agents have been searched according to their efficacy and specificity for glioma imaging in research centers and clinics.

MRI Agents for Glioma Imaging

Apart from routinely used MRI techniques, improved MRI techniques exhibit higher potential in evaluating the pathological features and grading of gliomas before the treatment [53]. The cellularity of gliomas has been evaluated by either T2-weighted MR images or diffusion-weighted imaging (DWI) detecting free water molecular diffusion. DWI can be used for the differentiation of tumor necrosis from the abscess cavity especially for research purposes [54, 55]. Contrast agents comprising Gadolinium (Gd) chelates are generally used for glioma imaging by MRI. However, due to limited stability of Gd based contrast agents in circulation and the risk of formation of renal fibrosis, chelated forms of Gd, nanoparticular based iron oxide particles, and multifunctional MRI contrast agents have also been searched [56].

Gadolinium

Gd, a paramagnetic heavy metal, has a high ratio among MRI contrast agents. Due to the high toxicity of free gadolinium ion (Gd^{+3}), it is generally applied in chelated form for reducing its toxicity and enhancing body clearance. Chelators can be linear or macrocyclic [57]. A study related to the evaluation of Gd accumulation in brain tumor biopsy was performed on 28 patients by visual inspection and Scanning Electron Microscopy-Energy Dispersive X-Ray Spectroscopy (SEM-EDS). These accumulation sites are generally found with the contribution of calcification in high-grade vascular tumor sites [58]. In another study performed by Kiviniemi *et al.*, Gd was accumulated not only in live tumor tissues but also in neighboring normal brain tissues and necrotic tissues [59].

The position of Gd atom(s) is essential for contrast enhancement of gadolinium-based contrast agents. Single- and multi-arm ("star") Gd conjugates as antibody- and peptide-targeted nanosized contrast agents (NCAs) were synthesized by using polymalic acid platforms of different sizes [60]. Glioma imaging potential of these contrast agents was evaluated on human U87MG xenografts as glioma models after administration. Targeted NCAs having star-PEG features exhibited better relaxivity and greater contrast compared with commercial MultiHance contrast agents. Another study was performed by Fonchy *et al.* [61] for the design of a new Gd-based contrast agent which is called P760. For this purpose, the C6 rat glioma model was used to characterize brain tumor heterogeneity and image vascularization. Although Gd concentration was five times smaller in P760 than Gd-DOTA, similar contrast enhancement was observed for both agents.

Some novel MRI contrast agents have been searching for evaluating *in vivo* levels of other angiogenic proteins that are over-expressed in malignant brain tumors such as vascular endothelial growth factor receptor 2 (VEGF-R2) [62, 63], tumor cell migration/invasion marker, such as c-Met, a tyrosine kinase receptor for the scatter factor (hepatocyte growth factor) [64, 65], and inflammatory marker, inducible nitric oxide synthase (iNOS) [66, 67]. A study was performed by He *et al*, for evaluating the effectiveness of Gd-DTPA-albumin-anti-VEGFR2-biotin probe in the detection of regional differences in VEGFR2 levels *in vivo* in a C6 glioma model, and probe-specificity for glioma tissue by MRI [62]. It was observed that Gd-DTPA-albumin-anti-VEGFR2-biotin probe gave better results than non-targeted ones in glioma imaging.

Super Paramagnetic Iron Oxide Nanoparticles

Nanotechnology has been used for targeting of diseases effectively for effective diagnosis and imaging of several diseases. Enhanced resolution and sensitivity can be obtained by the use of nanocarriers in MRI to obtain accurate anatomical images. Due to long half-life and small particle size, superparamagnetic iron oxide nanoparticles (SPIONs) are one of the most frequently searched MRI contrast agents [68]. Additionally, particle size, surface properties, coating, and surface charge of iron oxide nanoparticles (IONPs) can be altered according to the desired scope and imaging disease site [69, 70].

IONPs have been searched as potential MRI contrast agents for imaging of glioma and intracranial neoplasms in brain tissue. PEG-coated IONPs designated enhanced circulation time, glioma targeting, and tumor accumulation due to the EPR effect [71]. SPIONs have been searched pretty much due to several advantages such as high sensitivity, non-toxicity, and bioavailability [72].

Lactoferrin is a type of transferrin and can enhance BBB penetration. Lactoferrin conjugated SPIONs have been developed by Xie *et al*. [72]. Transferrin receptors such as LRP1 are highly expressed in many cancer types including breast, ovarian, and brain cancers like glioma. Lf-SPIONs designated very little cytotoxicity. While T2-weighted images exhibited a stable contrast enhancement 48 h postinjection in glioma, surrounding tissues showed very little contrast enhancement. Therefore, Lf-SPIONs found potential as MRI contrast imaging agents for glioma diagnosis, imaging, image-guided surgery, and monitoring the efficacy of radiotherapy [72 - 76].

Both Gd- and iron oxide-based contrast agents were also developed in some studies to characterize c-Met levels in C6 gliomas. c-Met, a tumor marker, is over-expressed in many malignant cancers. It is a kind of indication of tumor invasiveness. The distribution of c-Met was found to be mainly concentrated in peri-tumor regions [64, 65, 77].

SPECT Agents for Glioma Imaging

When compared with PET tracers, SPECT tracers can be obtained easier and cheaper. However, their limited specificity and spatial resolution are some of the disadvantages. Additionally, the use of collimators causes a significant reduction in detection and diagnostic efficacy. $^{99m}TcO_4^-$, ^{99m}Tc- diethylenetriaminepentaacetic acid (^{99m}Tc-DTPA), ^{99m}Tc-hexamethylpropyleneamine oxime (^{99m}Tc-HMPAO), ^{99m}Tc-ethylene cysteine dimer (^{99m}Tc-ECD), ^{99m}Tc-methoxyisobutyl isonitrile (^{99m}Tc-MIBI), ^{99m}Tc-Tetrofosmin, ^{123}I-alpha-methyl-L-tyrosine (^{123}I-IMT), ^{111}In-Pentetreotide, Thallium-201 Chloride (^{201}Tl), and ^{67}Ga-citrate are SPECT radiopharmaceuticals used for imaging of brain tumors due to the mechanism of enhanced metabolic activity and altered BBB penetration. Among these tracers ^{201}Tl, ^{99m}Tc-MIBI and ^{123}I-IMT are generally used and searched agents for glioma imaging by SPECT [78].

Thallium-201 Chloride

^{201}Tl scintigraphy provides high accuracy in the grading of brain tumors. Images can be obtained 20-30 min. after *i.v.* injection of 2-5 mCi ^{201}Tl-chloride by gamma scintigraphy or SPECT. In a study performed by Ancri *et al.*, 1.5-2 mCi ^{201}Tl was given to the patients having cerebral lesions such as gliomas, meningiomas, metastases, infarctions, hematoms, hypophysis adenomas, and the results were compared with the patients administered 10-15 mCi ^{99m}Tc-pertechnetate. Lesions were accurately detected with ^{201}Tl which was found more effective than ^{99m}Tc-pertechnetate [78]. It was also observed that there is a good correlation between cellular proliferation and ^{201}Tl uptake [79]. However, ^{201}Tl has a limited utilization in routine applications when compared with ^{99m}Tc labeled radiopharmaceuticals due to its higher physical half-life (73 h.), lower energy photons, and lower radiation characteristics (69-80 keV). Another study was performed by Soricelli *et al.* to evaluate and compare the feasibility of brain tumors by ^{99m}Tc-tetrofosmin and ^{201}Tl SPECT. A significant relationship was observed between T/B ratios of ^{201}Tl and ^{99m}Tc-tetrofosmin. T/B ratio of ^{99m}Tc-tetrofosmin was found significantly higher than that of ^{201}Tl. While, both tracers exhibited high tumor accumulation, ^{99m}Tc-tetrofosmin designated tumor borders accurately. It was concluded that ^{99m}Tc-tetrofosmin was found better in the differentiation of brain tumors with a better definition of tumor margins [80].

^{99m}Tc-MIBI

10-30 mCi doses of ^{99m}Tc-MIBI was administered to 19 children by Treves *et al.* for brain tumor imaging and comparing the results with ^{201}Tl. Both agents exhibited similar accumulation. Sixty-seven percent sensitivity for both ^{201}Tl and ^{99m}Tc-MIBI, 91% specificity for ^{201}Tl, and 100% specificity for ^{99m}Tc-MIBI were observed. It was reported that lesion limits were detected better with ^{99m}Tc-MIBI and found parallel with ^{201}Tl [81]. In another study performed by Soler *et al.*

^{99m}Tc–MIBI was evaluated in 35 high-grade glioma patients for tumor recurrence. ^{99m}Tc-MIBI designated a fine differentiation of tumor recurrence from radiation necrosis [82]. In another study, the uptake of ^{99m}Tc-MIBI and ^{201}Tl was compared in 25 patients having malignant brain tumors. It was observed that ^{99m}Tc-MIBI can differentiate malignant brain tumors similar to ^{201}Tl. ^{99m}Tc-MIBI exhibited clearer identification of boundaries than ^{201}Tl in malignant brain tumors. However, the prediction of histological diagnosis using ^{99m}Tc-MIBI was not superior to ^{201}Tl [83].

^{123}*I-Alpha-Methyl-Tyrosine*

^{123}I-IMT is an emerging SPECT agent in tumor imaging. ^{123}I-IMT is an alternative SPECT imaging agent to more expensive PET tracers such as ^{11}C-MET. The first study related to the uptake of this tracer was performed in the late 1980s by Biersack *et al.* and significant contrast enhancement was observed in tumor tissue of 9 of 10 glioma patients [84].

In a study performed by Kuwert *et al*, ^{123}I-IMT accumulation was evaluated in 53 patients (40 patients having varying levels of glioma and 13 patients having neoplastic lesions). ^{123}I-IMT designated 71% sensitivity and 83% specificity in the differentiation of low leveled gliomas. ^{123}I-IMT also designated 82% sensitivity and 100% specificity in the differentiation of high-grade gliomas from non-neoplastic lesions. However, non-neoplastic lesions could not be successfully differentiated from low-grade gliomas [85]. In another study performed by the same group, IMT was found successful in the differentiation of glioma recurrence and radiation necrosis with 78% sensitivity and 100% specificity [86]. IMT-SPECT and FDG-PET were compared by Weber *et al.* in a group of patients. IMT was found more reliable than FDG in tumor detection and tumor size evaluation [87].

PET Agents for Glioma Imaging

PET has been successfully used for glioma imaging by the use of proper and specific positron-emitting radiopharmaceuticals. Biopsy guiding, diagnosing primary brain tumor, directing of radiotherapy and distinguishing between tumor recurrence and radionecrosis after initial therapy can be achieved by the use of proper PET tracers. For this purpose, several positron-emitting radionuclides including ^{18}F, ^{11}C, ^{13}N, and ^{15}O can be used for radiolabeling of proper specific ligands. A table of positron-emitting radionuclides, half-life, production method, and energy is given (Table **1**).

Table 1. Positron emitting radionuclides and their half-life, production method, and energy.

Radionulide	Half-life	Production Method	Emax (MeV)
C-11	20 min.	$^{10}B(d,n)^{11}C$ $^{14}N(p,\alpha)^{11}C$	0.3856
N-13	10 min.	$^{12}C(d,n)^{13}N$ $^{16}O(p,\alpha)^{13}N$ $^{13}C(p,n)^{13}N$	1,19
O-15	2 min.	$^{14}N(d,n)^{15}O$ $^{15}N(p,n)^{15}O$	0,97
F-18	110 min.	$^{18}O(p,n)^{18}F$	0,635
Cu-64	13 h.	$^{63}Cu(n,\gamma)^{64}Cu$ $^{64}Zn(n,p)^{64}Cu$ $^{64}Ni(p,n)^{64}Cu$	0.66
Zr-89	79 h.	$^{89}Y(p,n)^{89}Zr$	0.89
Sc-44	238 min.	$^{44}Ti/^{44}Sc$ generator	0,632
Rb-82	1,3 min.	$^{82}Sr/^{82}Rb$ generator	3.378
Ga-68	68 min.	$^{68}Ge/^{68}Ga$ generator $^{68}Zn(p,n)^{68}Ga$	1,89
I-124	100 h.	$^{124}Te(p,n)^{124}I$	1.535
Y-86	15 h.	$^{86}Sr(p,n)^{86}Y$	1.221
Br-76	16 h.	$As(3He,2n)^{76}Br$	3.382

^{18}F-Fluorodeoxyglucose (^{18}F-FDG) is one of the widely used PET tracers in oncology [88]. However, it is not a specific radiopharmaceutical for intracranial use. Therefore, more specific and sensitive radiotracers exist which can target different metabolic pathways and functions of glioma. Cell division was induced and cell division rate was enhanced in all tumoral tissues. Therefore, protein and DNA synthesis and glycolysis were also enhanced simultaneously [50]. The use of specific radiocontrast agents for the detection of these mechanisms can provide better diagnosis and differentiation. Different novel and more specific tracers have been searched for glioma imaging, grading, and therapy response. Although most of these novel PET tracers were found to be more specific for accurate diagnosis of glioma when compared to FDG-PET, ^{18}F-FDG remains as the routine application option in clinics. Currently, most of these novel PET tracers stayed at the research level.

Glycolysis: ^{18}F-FDG

FDG is ^{18}F-labeled glucose and it is taken by the cells with a mechanism similar to glucose in physiological conditions and stays till metabolization. ^{18}F-FDG PET imaging is generally used for the detection of systemic cancers [89]. The expression of glucose transporters and FDG uptake were enhanced by the induction of glycolysis. Therefore, FDG-PET provides the evaluation of *in vivo* glycolysis metabolism [89].

^{18}F-FDG-PET can be used for tumor grading, monitoring of therapy response, and differentiation of primary brain tumors from radiation necrosis [52, 88]. ^{18}F-FDG was found more successful in the differentiation of high-grade gliomas from other brain tumors and especially in the primary diagnosis of gliomas compared to MRI [90].

However, as it is widely known, ^{18}F-FDG-PET has some limitations in the characterization of brain tumors due to the high glucose metabolic rate of the brain. Apart from high-grade tumors, many tumors designate lesser or equal signals with brain tissue [52]. Additionally, ^{18}F-FDG accumulation is affected by many factors including membrane glucose transport protein (GLUT-1) mediated accumulation, hypoxic formations, enhancement of vessel intensity, and oncogene activation [91].

Protein Synthesis: Aminoacid Tracers (^{11}C-MET and ^{18}F-FET)

Enhanced protein synthesis and amino acid transport in glioma cells have been led the utilization of radiolabeled amino acid tracers in glioma imaging since 1982 [92]. Studies comparing radiolabeled amino acid tracers and ^{18}F-FDG in the evaluation of brain tumors designated that tumor contrast was observed accurately with higher sensitivity by the application of radiolabeled amino acid tracers [91].

The accumulation of radiolabeled amino acid tracers in normal brain tissue is lesser than ^{18}F-FDG. Therefore, radiolabeled amino acid tracers provide the differentiation of small tumors from normal tissues. ^{11}C-MET, ^{18}F-FET, ^{18}F-FDOPA have been used for research purposes and also in clinics [80]. These radiolabeled amino acid tracers are the reason for the choice in neuro-oncology [51, 93]. One of the most significant advantages of radiolabeled amino acid tracers is high tumor accumulation even when BBB is intact [50]. Although these amino acid radiotracers are not FDA approved in the United States currently, they have been used as a standard of care in Europe and other parts of the world with numerous studies [94, 95].

[11]C-MET

One of the most commonly used radiolabeled amino acid tracers in brain tumor imaging is ^{11}C-MET. ^{11}C-MET has a physical half-life of 20 min. and it has been widely used and searched in many centers as being an ^{11}C-labeled amino acid since the 1980s. Due to the short half-life of ^{11}C, ^{18}F-labeled amino acid analogs were also developed.

[11]C-MET is an analog of essential amino acid and it is used in protein synthesis. Due to significantly higher uptake of methionine in tumor tissue, the tumor can be accurately and simply imaged by radiolabeled methionine [50].

It was observed in many studies that radiolabeled amino acid tracers gave better and trustable images when compared with ^{18}F-FDG [96 - 98]. In a study performed by Shinozaki *et al.* in 70 patients having intracerebral gliomas, ^{11}C-MET-PET designated a significant contribution to histological and preoperative findings in low-grade gliomas especially. It was observed that T/N ratio was enhanced significantly [99].

Molecular features such as isocitrate dehydrogenase (IDH) mutation have gained importance in glioma subtyping due to 2016 WHO classification. A pilot trial was performed for the evaluation of the potential of ^{11}C-MET PET/MRI in the classification of glioma according to the revised WHO classification using a machine learning model. For this purpose, MET-PET/MRI imaging was performed for WHO grade II–IV glioma patients. It was observed that MET-PET/MRI imaging was found useful for the detection of IDH in glioma patients [100]. Another similar study was performed by another group evaluating the relationship between the uptake of ^{11}C-MET, ^{11}C-CHO, and ^{18}F-FDG by PET imaging and IDH status (wild-type [IDH-wt] or mutant [IDH-mut]) in astrocytic and oligodendroglial tumors according to 2016 WHO classification. For this purpose, 105 cerebral glioma patients were evaluated. A significant difference was observed in T/N ratios for all PET tracers between IDH-wt and IDH-mut groups. MET-PET, CHO-PET, and FDG-PET were observed informative for differentiating IDH-wt and IDH-mut tumors in gliomas according to the 2016 WHO classification [101].

Ozaki *et al.* studied the validation of the quality of tumor segmentation with Brain Tumor Image Analysis (BraTumIA) in comparison with results obtained from ^{11}C-MET PET. BraTumIA is an automated segmentation tool for detecting brain tumors imaged by MRI. For this purpose, 45 high-grade glioma patients were imaged by MRI and MET-PET. It was observed that significantly higher underestimation and overestimation errors were obtained by calculation of BraTumIA than that of MET-PET [102].

Michaud *et al.* studied the diagnosis of recurrent gliomas with an ^{18}F-labeled synthetic analog of amino acid L-leucine (^{18}F-Fluciclovine) and compared its efficacy with MRI and ^{11}C-MET PET in brain tumor patients. Tumor uptake of ^{18}F-Fluciclovine exhibited good correlation with ^{11}C-MET but gave significantly higher image contrast [103].

In another study performed by Kato *et al.* in 95 glioma patients (37 grade II, 37 grade III and 21 grade IV), ^{11}C-MET, ^{18}F-FDG, and ^{11}C-Choline (CHO) were administered to evaluate the metabolic activity. Tumor localization was observed better with MET-PET than FDG-PET and CHO-PET [104]. In another study performed by Pirotte *et al.*, in 59 low grade and 23 high-grade glioma patients, MET-PET found effective in the differentiation and tumor volume detection of 88% low-grade tumors and 78% high-grade tumors [105]. Gumprecht *et al.* studied the role of preoperative evaluation of ^{11}C-MET-PET in low-grade gliomas. MET-PET found a good mediator in stereotaxic biopsy guiding in 20 low-grade patients [106, 107]. In another study, ^{11}C-MET was found better than ^{18}F-FDG in stereotactic biopsy guiding [90].

Ono *et al.* evaluated the efficacy of amino acid PET tracers ^{11}C-MET and trans-1-amino-3-18F-fluorocyclobutanecarboxylic acid (anti-^{18}F-FACBC) for detecting early responses to Temozolomide (TMZ), interferon-β (IFN), and Bevacizumab (Bev) combination therapies in glioblastoma. For this purpose, U87MG cells were incubated with low dose TMZ to induce chemoresistance before the administration of both anti-^{14}C-FACBC and ^{3}H-MET. The efficacy of single agent (TMZ, Bev) and combination therapy (TMZ/IFN, TMZ/Bev, TMZ/IFN/Bev) was evaluated in orthotopic gliomas. It was reported that, while TMZ and TMZ/IFN combination treatment decreased ^{3}H-thymidine (TdR) accumulation and the volume of distribution of anti-^{14}C-FACBC and ^{3}H-MET in U87 but not U87R cells, Bev did not exhibit any effect *in vitro*. *In vivo* results showed that TMZ therapy significantly decreased tracer accumulation and proliferation of U87, but not U87R-derived tumors. Bev treatment decreased U87 enhancing lesions significantly. Both TMZ/IFN and TMZ/IFN/Bev combination treatment decreased tracer accumulation and proliferation in U87R tumors significantly as well. The treatment response was evaluated poorly by MRI. It was observed that an effective treatment was achieved by TMZ/IFN/Bev which can be monitored effectively by PET with the use of amino acid tracers [108].

^{18}F-FET

^{18}F-FET is an amino acid analog that has been used since the 1990s. It has a sufficiently long half-life (110 min.) for imaging and monitoring of biodistribution. It was observed that ^{18}F-FET has taken the place of ^{11}C-MET in many neuro-oncology centers all around Europe in the last decade due to several advantages including higher *in vivo* stability, higher T/N ratio and especially longer half-life [93]. A study related to a convenient synthesis of ^{18}F-FET was performed by Hamacher *et al.* They synthesized ^{18}F-FET with a procedure to achieve a remotely controlled no-carrier-added and enantiomerically pure tracer. A radiochemical yield of 60% was obtained within 80 mins [109]. Another study related to ^{18}F-FET radiosynthesis was performed by Siddiq *et al.* Although ^{18}F-FET has some advantages in brain tumor imaging when compared with ^{18}F-FDG and ^{11}C-MET, it has some limitations in radiosynthesis and quality control. They performed a modification in ^{18}F-FET production by the use of a commercially

available fully automated GRP Scintomics module to handle the limitations and simplify the quality control procedure. It was reported that a high radiochemical and enantiomeric purity (more than 99%) was achieved in ^{18}F-FET production [110].

Although biopsy location, tumor description and recurrence detection of ^{18}F-FET and ^{11}C-MET are very similar [111], higher *in vivo* stability, faster uptake kinetics, lesser uptake in non-tumor tissues, easier synthesis protocol and higher half-life (110 min.) of ^{18}F-FET make it a desirable amino acid tracer when compared with ^{11}C-MET. Therefore, FET-PET provides essential information in the detection of biopsy boarders, cerebral glioma therapy planning, sensitive monitoring of therapy response, and differentiation of tumor recurrence from necrosis related to radiotherapy or combined chemotherapy [93, 112 - 116].

It was observed that L-enantiomer of FET is 24 times more stereoselective than D-enantiomer in the mouse brain [117]. Kaim *et al.* reported that FET designated higher specificity and lower accumulation in non-neoplastic inflammatory cells and inflammatory lymph nodes when compared to MET and FDG [118, 119]. Additionally, it was observed that FET accumulation was found lower in irradiated tumors, hematomas, and cerebral ischemia generally [120].

In another study performed on 14 patients having intracerebral lesions, diagnostic values of ^{18}F-FET and FDG-PET were evaluated. Although FET-PET found potential in the diagnosis of brain tumors, it was demonstrated limited specificity in the differentiation of neoplastic and non-neoplastic lesions similar to FDG-PET. Therefore, histopathological evaluation of biopsy samples was found beneficial according to the study [121].

While high-grade gliomas reached to the pick value at 10-15 min. after the injection of FET and following a decrease, low-grade gliomas or non-neoplastic lesions exhibited a retarded and constantly increasing FET uptake [122 - 124]. In a study performed on 462 patients, FET-PET exhibited 82% sensitivity and 76% specificity in the diagnosis of primary brain tumors [125]. In another study performed on 393 patients, FET-PET was found to be successful in the differentiation of neoplastic lesions from non-neoplastic ones with 87% sensitivity and 68% specificity [126].

^{18}F-FET uptake was observed 80% in Grade I, 79% in Grade II, 92% in Grade III, and 100% in Grade IV glioma patients according to WHO [126]. Therefore, it is thought that tumor grading can be performed due to FET uptake. It was also observed that oligodendroglial gliomas designated higher FET uptake when compared to astrocytomas due to higher cell density, different L-amino acid transporter systems, or higher microvessel density [127].

^{18}F-FLT which is a proliferation indicator can accumulate in cerebral gliomas depending on the degree of malignity. However, it can not penetrate through intact BBB [128]. On the contrary, altered BBB penetration is not a prerequisite for brain penetration of FET depending on the accumulation ability of neutral amino acids in brain tissue [120, 129]. Many studies were performed for the evaluation of the diagnostic value of ^{18}F-FET PET [130 - 134].

Amino Acid Analog: ^{18}F-DOPA

While ^{18}F-DOPA is an amino acid tracer to provide information related to the integrity of presynaptic dopaminergic pathways in Neurology, it is also accumulated in neuroendocrine tumors. FDOPA is taken by the cells in glial tumors by sodium-dependent amino acid transporter systems. It was reported that FDOPA gave information in the grading of recently diagnosed glial tumors and proliferation rates. Similar to ^{11}C-MET and ^{18}F-FET, ^{18}F-FDOPA also exhibited higher accumulation in high-grade tumors than low-grade ones [50].

In a study performed by Kratochwil *et al.*, the uptake of ^{18}F-FDOPA and ^{18}F-FET was compared in high-grade and low-grade recurrent glioma patients. ^{18}F-FDOPA exhibited earlier arrival to the peak value in both low and high-grade gliomas and higher tumor/blood (T/B) ratio compared to ^{18}F-FET [124, 135].

It was observed that the differentiation of tumor and necrosis was higher with ^{18}F-FDOPA PET compared to MRI. Although tumor volume was observed similar for both images, tumor infiltration degree was observed accurately higher with ^{18}F-FDOPA [136, 137]. In a study performed by Ledezme *et al.*, the combination of ^{18}F-FDOPA-PET and MRI gave higher accuracy in lesion detection [138]. Additionally, ^{18}F-FDOPA-PET was found effective in the differentiation of tumor recurrence from alterations related to therapy [139].

In a study comparing the uptake of ^{18}F-FET and ^{18}F-DOPA in high-grade gliomas, ^{18}F-FET exhibited higher SUV value and tumor/background (T/B) ratio [135]. Another study was performed to evaluate the value of dynamic ^{18}F-FDOPA PET parameters for predicting the molecular features of newly diagnosed gliomas. For this purpose, ^{18}F-FDOPA was applied to 58 patients to diagnose glioma according to the WHO 2016 classification. It was concluded that the prediction of molecular features of glioma was achieved by ^{18}F-FDOPA PET with dynamic uptake parameters [140].

DNA Synthesis: ^{18}F-FLT

DNA synthesis rate detection, which gives essential information about tumor malignancy and prognosis, is a target of many chemotherapeutic agents and molecular imaging probes. ^{18}F-FLT accumulation in the cell gives a clue about the activity of the tymidine kinaz-1 enzyme. Intact BBB is an obstacle for the accumulation of ^{18}F-FLT in brain tissue. On the other hand, ^{18}F-FLT was found successful in the evaluation of radiotherapy response and tumor recurrence when BBB was damaged [50, 92].

A study was performed for the evaluation of the combination of ^{18}F-FLT PET and MRI for the diagnosis of glioma and its comparison with MRI alone by correlating with histopathological features. For this purpose, 13 patients with a supratentorial malignant glioma were subjected to ^{18}F-FLT PET and MRI. During surgery, an average of 11 biopsies per patient was taken. It was observed that positive predictive value was 93.1% for MRI alone and 78.3% for combined MRI and PET. Additional tumoral tissue was detected by the combination of MRI and ^{18}F-FLT-PET in newly diagnosed glioma patients. Some results about the underestimation of the lesion margins were obtained by ^{18}F-FLT which were not correlated with the histopathological data [141].

In a study performed by Chen *et al.*, ^{18}F-FLT and ^{18}F-FDG were compared in the evaluation of high-grade gliomas. High uptake of ^{18}F-FLT was observed in high-grade tumor patients (grade III ve IV) especially. ^{18}F-FLT found better than ^{18}F-FDG in the evaluation of tumor prognosis [142].

Another study about the comparison of the ability of monitoring therapy efficacy by PET and MRI was performed by Corroyer-Dulmont *et al.* in recurrent glioblastoma multiforme model. To obtain PET images, ^{18}F-FDG and ^{18}F-FLT were administered after treatment to compare late tumor growth and survival. It was reported that treatment decreased tumor volume and increased survival. It was observed that the prediction of Temozolomide+Bevacizumab treatment efficacy was successfully observed with ^{18}F-FLT by PET/MRI [143].

Hypoxia: ^{18}F-FMISO

Enhancement in the metabolism synthesis functions of tumor cells causes an enhancement in the required energy and metabolites. Angiogenesis is induced to meet this requirement and oxygenation supply. Tumor hypoxia is formed due to rapid proliferation and on the contrary insufficient oxygenation. Hypoxia is related to peripheric growth of tumor, tumor progression, and radiotherapy resistance. It was observed that nitroimidazole derivative ^{18}F-FMISO and ^{18}F-FAZA were proper tracers for the evaluation of hypoxia [50, 92].

A multivariate model was performed in a study by using several MRI markers of blood flow, vascular permeability, and accumulation of ^{18}F-FDG to predict the extent of hypoxia in ^{18}F-FMISO positive regions. For this purpose, 27–74 years old fifteen patients with brain tumors (glioma, n = 13; lymphoma, n = 1; germinoma, n = 1) were subjected to MRI scans using a 3T scanner and dynamic contrast-enhanced (DCE) perfusion and arterial spin labeling images and PET scans were also obtained after the administration of ^{18}F-FDG and ^{18}F-FMISO. It was observed that by the use of a multivariate prediction model, the extent of hypoxia in FMISO-positive areas can be predicted in patients with brain tumors [144].

In a study performed by Cher *et al*, while ^{18}F-FMISO uptake was observed in high-grade glioma patients, it did not observe in low-grade glioma patients. ^{18}F-FMISO uptake was also observed in parallel with the expression of VEGFR1 and antigen Ki-67 [145]. In another study performed by Valk *et al.*, tumor uptake was observed accurately in high-grade glioma patients 5 min. after administration. It was observed that T/B contrast was reached to an equilibrium 40-50 min. after administration and tumor activity was reduced after that time. Therefore, it was concluded that ^{18}F-FMISO-PET scans should be performed shortly after the administration to evaluate the hypoxia in glioma [146].

Cell Membrane Synthesis: ^{11}C-CHO

Choline is an essential component of cell membrane phospholipids. Therefore, the level of this component is enhanced in rapidly proliferating tumor cells. It was designated that choline is accumulated in brain tumors and especially in high-grade lesions by MRI. ^{11}C-CHO uptake was observed better than ^{18}F-FDG in glioma patients [147]. In another study, MET-PET was observed superior when compared with FDG-PET and CHO-PET in visual inspection of tumor lesions [104].

Other Radioactive Tracers

More specific radiotracers have been searched recently due to the need for early and specific detection of glioma.

Radiolabeled RGD Agents

For this purpose, integrins have been searched as heterodimer transmembrane proteins which can bind to the molecules having arginine-glycine-aspartic acid (RGD) amino acid series. These series exist at extracellular matrix glycoproteins, the surface of some cells, and some complement proteins [148]. The use of radiolabeled biomolecules provides the detection of potential molecular alterations in tumor tissue similar to specific monoclonal antibodies and peptides.

Brain tumors are angiogenesis dependent on a high ratio. Cell adhesion receptor integrin $\alpha v\beta3$ is highly expressed in glioma and active endothelial cells which plays a significant role in brain tumor growth, expansion, and angiogenesis. Properly radiolabeled $\alpha v\beta3$ integrin-antagonists are used in the imaging of angiogenesis-related brain tumors [149]. For this purpose, RGD peptides are recently searched for PET integrin imaging by radiolabeling with a proper PET radionuclide such as ^{68}Ga or ^{18}F. Especially cyclic or linear RGD peptides are searched for molecular imaging of expression degree of the cell membrane, tumor angiogenesis, proliferation, and therapy effectiveness after radiolabeling by a metal chelator such as DOTA [150, 151].

Integrin $\alpha v\beta_3$ was highly expressed in both neovascular and glioma cells. ^{68}Ga-PRGD$_2$ has been searched as a novel glioma imaging agent. It was observed as a specific agent in the detection of neovascular formation and glioma grading [152].

^{68}Ga-aquibeprin and ^{68}Ga-avebetrin are PET tracers for selective imaging and mapping of integrins $\alpha5\beta1$ and $\alpha v\beta3$, respectively. Notni *et al.* investigated the specific activity of both tracers on *in vivo* imaging. The highest tumor/tissue ratio was achieved in *ex vivo* biodistribution and PET imaging for comparably large doses like 6 nmol ^{68}Ga-aquibeprin per mouse (3.5 MBq/nmol). Therefore, ^{68}Ga-aquibeprin and ^{68}Ga-avebetrin perform selective imaging of target sites having different integrin expression levels by adjusting specific activity [153].

^{18}F-labeled glycosylated RGD peptide ^{18}F-Galacto-RGD was observed successfully in imaging of integrin $\alpha_v\beta_3$ expression related to tumor-related angiogenesis [92]. Glycosylation of this peptide provides an alteration of pharmacokinetics profile and higher tumor accumulation. Radiolabeling of this peptide was performed by 4-nitrophenyl-2-^{18}F-fluoropropionate. ^{18}F-Galacto-RGD was synthesized with 85% of radiochemical efficiency and higher than 98% of radiochemical purity [154].

In a study performed by Schnell *et al*, ^{18}F-Galacto-RGD designated high accumulation in the area of highly proliferating glial tumor cells with a high SUV which was found parallel with immunohistochemical $\alpha v\beta_3$ integrin expression. Therefore, this tracer was evaluated as a promising one especially in therapy planning and monitoring [155].

Antisense Oligonucleotides

Antisense oligonucleotides (ASO) are small nucleic acid chains having the ability to bind cellular RNA by a hybridization mechanism. Binding of molecules having an antisense effect on specific mRNA prevents the expression of related genes. Synthetic oligonucleotides exhibit antisense effect [156, 157]. The use of radiolabeled antisense oligonucleotides provides a deep approach for enlightening *in vivo* tumor biochemistry and the development of novel radiotracers for glioma imaging. The use of antisense oligonucleotides is beneficial depending on providing visualization and targeting the expression of specific mRNA, protein expression, and an endogenous gene [92].

The use of antisense oligonucleotides as diagnostic agents is very attractive nowadays. Antisense oligonucleotides are used for not only monitoring of active genes but also preventing peptide synthesis by hybridization to mRNA series in the cells. Therefore, these oligonucleotides are thought to be proper molecules for the therapy of diseases. The use of antisense oligonucleotides as *in vivo* imaging agents has some disadvantages including radiosynthesis, stability, targeting, and binding abilities which may be improved by research [158, 159].

A study was performed by Hnatowich *et al.* about the development of hydrazine nicotinamide-^{99m}Tc chelates (SHNH) for the radiolabeling of DNA. About 60% of radiolabeling efficiency was obtained [160].

^{111}In is another proper radionuclide for the development of antisense oligonucleotide probes due to long half-life (2.8 days) which is proper for long biodistribution of antisense oligonucleotides [161]. A study was performed by Fujibayashi *et al.* for the synthesis of a new ^{111}In labeled antisense probe. Radiolabeling efficiency of isothiocyanobenzyl-EDTA (IBE) conjugated oligonucleotide was found higher than 90% [162]. ^{123}I and ^{125}I isotopes were used as SPECT antisense imaging due to proper physical half-lives and energies [163, 164].

PET radionuclides were also tried for antisense oligonucleotide radiolabeling. ^{18}F was successfully used for radiolabeling of antisense oligonucleotides due to its proper half-life (110 min.) and high energy positron emission (0.6335 MeV) [164]. Another PET radionuclide ^{11}C is generally not proper for the radiolabeling of antisense oligonucleotides due to its short half-life (20 mins). However, some strategies have been tried to overcome this limitation [165, 166].

Due to the availability of ^{68}Ge/^{68}Ga generators, the use of ^{68}Ga as a PET radiotracer has been enhanced as an alternative to ^{18}F. Roivaienen *et al.* used DOTA as the macrocyclic chelating ligand for radiolabeling of antisense oligonucleotides with ^{68}GaCl$_3$. It was observed that ^{68}GaCl$_3$ was labeled to DOTA conjugated oligonucleotides easily and rapidly in 10 min. at 100°C. The radiochemical purity was found 99% after 30 min. of labeling and specific activity was observed about 68 mCi/μmole. It was reported that the use of DOTA chelator for ^{68}Ga labeling did not alter the hybridization of oligonucleotides or protein binding capacities [167].

Nanocarriers for Glioma Imaging

Drug delivery systems can deliver drugs and/or radiocontrast/contrast agents to the desired target tissue/organ within the body. In this way, improved efficacy and safety can be achieved for the diagnosis, imaging and/or therapy of the diseases. Improved diagnosis and/or therapy can be managed by surface modification, targeting, release modification, localization of drug delivery systems [168 - 170]. Drug delivery systems having a particle size less than 100 nm are generally called as nanocarriers. Nanosized delivery systems having a hydrophilic surface coating can generally escape from rapid clearance by macrophages within RES and can be benefited from the EPR effect to accumulate in the tumor site. Nanocarriers can be protected against plasma protein adsorption by a hydrophilic surface coating such as PEG, poloxamines, poloxamers, polysaccharides or branched, or block copolymers [46, 171, 172]. The physicochemical properties of some nanocarriers are given in Fig. (3) [173, 174].

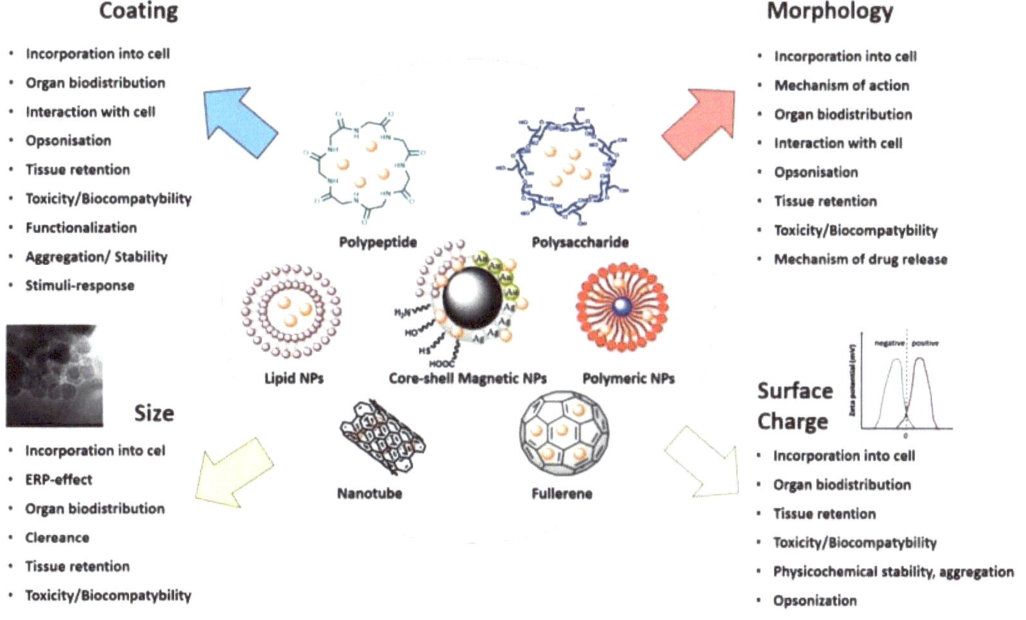

Fig. (3). Physicochemical features of some nanocarriers [173, 174].

For this purpose, PEG covalently linked to amphiphilic copolymers (polylactic acid, polycaprolactone, and polycyanoacrylate) have generally been chosen due to the ability to prevent aggregation and ligand desorption in blood components [172, 175, 176]. Other factors affecting drug release triggering at the tumor site include pH, redox potential, and tumor-activated prodrug therapy which may be benefitted for effective therapy [46, 177 - 179].

Enormous research and development have been performed in the field of brain cancer research especially on brain imaging, diagnosis, imaging-assisted surgeries, targeted drug delivery system based treatment, and adjuvant therapies. However, mortality related to brain cancers especially glioblastoma is still so high. Therefore, novel and effective diagnostic and imaging approaches are essentially needed as well as effective therapeutic approaches. In this concept, target-specific imaging agents and nanocarrier based approaches have been searched for effective imaging and diagnosis of glioma due to numerous advantages including reduced volume of distribution, protection of the content from enzymatic degradation or rapid removal from the circulation by RES, targeting of the disease site, enhancing target accumulation by specific ligand functionalization, longer circulation time, and toxicity reduction when compared to conventional agents [46]. A variety of nanocarriers exist for the design of novel imaging and/or therapy purposes of different diseases including glioma. These nanocarriers can be simply classified as; 1. polymeric nanocarriers (polymeric nanoparticles, polymeric micelles, dendrimers, polymer-drug conjugates, polymeric hydrogels, *etc.*), 2. lipid-based nanocarriers (liposomes, solid lipid nanoparticles, phospholipids, nanoemulsions, self-emulsifying drug delivery systems, *etc.*) and 3. inorganic nanocarriers (magnetic nanoparticles, gold nanoparticles, quantum dots, silica nanoparticles, carbon nanotubes, *etc.*) [180].

Molecular imaging benefiting from genetic features of the tumor would be of great value due to different characteristics of each tumor. Therefore, the use of target-specific nanoparticle-based imaging probes has to be designed for glioma diagnosis and imaging. The use of targeted multifunctional nanoparticles for tumor diagnosis, imaging, and staging could provide enhanced contrast for specific and effective detection of tumor border and extent even at an earlier stage. This may also avoid unnecessary biopsy [46]. A variety of research has been performed for defining the importance of nanocarriers in specific and accurate imaging of glioma by different imaging modalities. A proper gamma or positron-emitting radionuclide, an MRI contrast agent, a CT contrast agent, a fluorescent dye, a NIR agent dye, or their combination can be encapsulated or labeled to nanocarrier based imaging radiocontrast or contrast agents to develop novel specific agents for glioma diagnosis and imaging.

A study was designed for the development of neuropilin-1 (NRP-1) targeted polypeptide tLyP-1 containing USPIO-PEG-tLyP-1 probe for imaging of glioma by MRI. USPIO-PEG-tLyP-1 was observed as an effective imaging probe for high and low-grade gliomas having different NRP-1 expression levels in glioma model nude mice injected U87 and CHG-5 cells [181].

The biological effect of RGD–labeled USPIO was investigated on human umbilical vein endothelial cells (HUVECs), ovarian carcinoma (MLS) cells, and glioblastoma cells (U87MG) and U87MG xenografts *in vivo*. It was observed that while RGD-USPIOs designated higher HUVECs and MLS cell accumulation than unspecific ones, RGD-USPIOs designated lesser U87MG cell internalization than USPIOs. Furthermore, free RGD and $\alpha v \beta 3$ integrin–blocking antibodies strongly reduced the endocytosis of nonspecific USPIOs only in U87MG cells. Additionally, RGD-USPIOs designated an accumulation only at the neovasculature of U87MG tumors which caused a significantly higher change in R2 relaxation rate of tumors than that of USPIOs [182].

Yang *et al.* prepared hybrid SiO_2 coated, Lactoferrin (Lf) receptor targeted, magnetite $NaGdF_4:Yb^{3+},Er^{3+},Li^+@NaGdF_4$ (UCNPs) (UCNPs@SiO2-CX-Lf) core-shell nanoparticles for dual Upconversion Luminescence (UCL) imaging and MRI. It was observed that UCNPs@SiO2-CX-Lf exhibited fine characteristics and BBB penetration in the tumor xenograft rat model by giving bright UCL signal and T1 MRI contrast [183].

The use of SPIONs, as nanoparticular based contrast agents, can enhance circulation time, efficiency, and prevent agglomeration. Graphene derivatives such as graphene oxide (GO) and reduced graphene oxide (RGO) are other delivery systems having both high surface area and functional moieties. Llenas *et al.* developed a simple, fast, and safe microwave-assisted approach for the synthesis of SPION-RGO hybrids. SPION-RGO hybrids were obtained with a very small particle size (7.1 nm) and homogeneous size distribution. These nanoparticles designated good relaxivity (r2*) values to obtain fine MR images and safe profiles at *in vitro* toxicity studies in GL261 glioma and J774 macrophage-like cells for 24 h [49].

Synthesized hybrid chitosan-dextran (CS-DX) SPIONs were prepared by Shevtsov *et al.* and characterized by transmission electron microscopy (TEM) and relaxometry studies. The characterization of CS-DX-SPIONs was found to be proper. The addition of chitosan increased the charge of the dextran-based SPIONs from +8.9 to +19.3 mV. Chitosan-based nanoparticles exhibited enhanced internalization in U87, C6 glioma, and HeLa cells than that of dextran-coated particles due to the results of confocal microscopy and flow cytometry studies. Both synthesized SPIONs designated an acceptable toxicity profile (10 µg/ml). CS-DX-SPIONs were observed to accumulate in the tumor site of orthotopic C6 gliomas in rats allowing improved tumor imaging [184].

For tumor prognosis and therapy, SPION-labeled C6 cells were used to monitor the migration by MRI. Satisfactory distribution and cell labeling were achieved by SPIONs at *in vitro* studies. SPION-induced T2- and T2*-weighted MRI signal reductions were achieved within the lesion [185].

Another study was performed by Moffat *et al.* related to the development of PEGylated, SPIO encapsulated nanoparticles for MRI of glioma cells. This polyacrylamide (PAM) SPIONs provided a significant T2 and T2* relaxivity. Additionally, these nanoparticles designated an enhanced plasma half-life and tumor uptake by MRI in rats bearing orthotopic 9L gliomas. Therefore, these PAM SPIONs may be used to image glioma resection [186, 187].

DTPA derivatized, PEGylated lipid-based nanoparticles were radiolabeled with different radiometals, including ^{111}In and ^{99m}Tc for SPECT imaging, ^{68}Ga for PET imaging, and ^{177}Lu for therapeutic applications. For this purpose, different DTPA amounts, compositions, and buffers were used. ^{99m}Tc-labeling was performed directly by $[^{99m}Tc(H_2O)_3(CO)_3]^+$. High labeling yields (>90%) were achieved for all radionuclides and different liposomal formulations. The highest specific activities were achieved for ^{111}In (>4 MBq/µg liposome). Additionally, the highest stability was achieved toward DTPA/histidine in serum (>80% RCP, 24 h. post preparation). It was observed that while the biodistribution of different radionuclides in Lewis rats was different, any significant difference was not observed between nanoparticles. Lower blood and liver retention were achieved with ^{99m}Tc and ^{68}Ga labeled nanoparticles compared to ^{111}In labeled ones. PEGylated DTPA comprising nanoparticles was evaluated suitable for high radiolabeling efficiency and targeting applications [188].

^{68}Ga radiolabeled, Gd-containing AGuIX@NODAGA nanoparticles were developed for PET/MRI. Nanoparticles were labeled with ^{68}Ga with high efficiency. It was observed that ^{68}Ga-AGuIX@NODAGA was accumulated passively in U87MG human glioblastoma tumor xenografts. ^{68}Ga-AGuIX@NODAGA remained stable at least 60 min postinjection. ^{68}Ga-AGuIX@NODAGA can be used as a dual-modality PET/MRI agent which can also be used for image-guided radiation therapy [189].

Gd-based nanoparticles (GBN-4Si/Gd) were formulated for MRI and therapy as radiosensitizing agents of brain tumors in healthy rats and rats grafted with 9L gliosarcoma tumors. These nanoparticles were radiolabeled with ^{111}In to achieve biodistribution data. It was observed that these Gd-based nanoparticles were accumulated in brain tumors of the rat brain [190].

High-grade glioma is generally associated with high infiltration of myeloid cells (TAMCs). TAMCs can be used as emerging therapeutic targets due to the suppression of antitumor immune responses and the promotion of tumor cell growth. Depending on integrin CD11b is being one of the highest expressed cell surface marker of TAMCs, Nigam *et al.* evaluated Zr-89 labeled anti-CD11b antibody (Ab) by DFO chelator for PET imaging of TAMCs in a syngeneic orthotopic mouse glioma model. Biodistribution study was conducted with or without a blocking dose of anti-CD11b Ab after 72 h post-injection of [^{89}Zr]anti-CD11b Ab. To validate the presence of CD11b+TAMCs, flow cytometry, and immunohistochemistry studies of dissected GL261 tumors were performed. It was observed that [^{89}Zr]anti-CD11b Ab immunoPET targeting CD11b+ cells (TAMCs) with a high specificity can be used in a mouse model of GBM [191].

Recently, Near-IR fluorescence (NIRF) imaging has been popularly searched for imaging of diseases especially tumors in preclinical studies for imaging and clinical image-guided oncological surgery. Several dyes have been searched for effective imaging. IR780 is one of the most frequently searched dyes having high tumor targeting and imaging potential. However, its hydrophobic property limits its clinical use. Li *et al.* prepared and characterized IR 780 encapsulated liposomes and phospholipid micelles for fluorescent imaging of malignant brain tumors. Both formulations exhibited accumulation in mitochondria *in vitro*. IR780-phospholipid micelles designated higher intra-tumoral accumulation than IR780-liposomes in U87MG ectopic tumors and intracranial tumor accumulation and potent NIRF signal intensity in glioma orthotopic models [192]. Zhou *et al.* developed a NIR dye IRDye 800CW labeled glucose analog, 2-deoxyglucose (2-DG), for *in vivo* optical imaging of orthotopic glioma in a mouse model. Significantly higher signal intensity was obtained from the tumoral tissue of the brain by dynamic fluorescence imaging. *Ex vivo* fluorescence imaging of the tumor-bearing whole-brain showed distinct tumor margins. Cytoplasmic locations of 2-DG dye were observed in tumor cells in detailed microscopic imaging [193].

Another and one of the most frequently searched NIR agent is indocyanine green (ICG). ICG is desired for its fine light absorption which is also efficient for laser-mediated photothermal therapy. It can be used as a multifunctional probe due to optical imaging and photothermal abilities. However, poor aqueous stability and concentration-dependent aggregation are some of the most important drawbacks. Folic acid and integrin αvβ3 monoclonal antibody (mAb) conjugated ICG-P--PEG nanoprobes were formulated. The interactions between amphiphilic ICG and PL-PEG were analyzed using absorption and fluorescence spectroscopy. The target specificity of dual-targeted nanoprobes was checked *via* laser scanning confocal microscope and flow cytometry by using different cell lines having different levels of folate receptors or integrin αvβ3 expression. It was observed that these stable folic acid and αvβ3 conjugated ICG-PL-PEG nanoprobes found potential for optical imaging and photothermal therapy of cancer [194].

Chlorotoxin modified, PEGylated, NIR molecule Cy5.5 comprising iron oxide nanoparticles were developed by Veiseh *et al.* for imaging of glioma cells by MRI and fluorescence microscopy. Significant uptake of nanoparticles by glioma cells was observed by both MRI and fluorescence microscopy [195].

Another study was performed related to the development of IRDye® 800CW encapsulated Phosphatidylserine (PS)-targeted liposomal nanoprobes for tumor imaging. These liposomes were functionalized with F(ab')2 fragments of PGN635 binding to PS. After the administration of liposomal formulations, tumor imaging can be accomplished by *in vivo* dynamic NIR imaging. Enhanced tumor/normal contrast was observed after irradiation of tumors to increase PS exposure. Additionally, distinct biodistribution and pharmacokinetics were achieved with PGN-L-800CW when compared with 800CW-PGN probes [196].

For the therapy of different types of tumors, photodynamic therapy (PDT) is getting an emerging option. PDT agent is generally accumulated in tumor tissue selectively and tumor imaging can also be accomplished. Its vascular effect is generally responsible for tumor eradication. Benachour *et al.* developed multifunctional NRP-1 peptide conjugated for vascular targeting, Gd labeled with DOTA and chlorin as photosensitizer comprising polysiloxane theranostic nanoparticles. It was observed that the nanoparticles preserved photophysical properties of encapsulated photosensitizer and exhibited photosensitivity to MDA-MB-231 cancer cells. The binding ability of multifunctional nanoparticles was assessed by targeting NRP-1 recombinant protein. PDT activity of multifunctional nanoparticles was assessed *in vitro* and it was evaluated that nanoparticles induced photocytotoxicity depending on the concentration of the photosensitizer molecules and light dose. A significant MRI contrast enhancement was achieved in tumor tissue of rats bearing intracranial U87 glioblastoma after the administration of multifunctional theranostic nanoparticles [197].

Another research was performed for developing MB encapsulated nanoparticles for imaging and PDT of the tumor. For this purpose, three different nanoparticles were developed including Polyacrylamide, sol-gel silica, and organically modified silicate (ORMOSIL) nanoparticles. After inducing by light irradiation, the amount of generated $^1O_2$ by entrapped MB was measured quantitatively with anthracene-9,10-dipropionic acid, and disodium salt was used to compare the effects of different matrices. While polyacrylamide nanoparticles designated the most efficient delivery of $^1O_2$, sol-gel nanoparticles had the best MB loading among other nanoparticles. To evaluate the matrix effect, *in vitro* PDT test was performed on rat C6 glioma cells with MB loaded polyacrylamide nanoparticles. Positive photodynamic results were observed with MB loaded polyacrylamide nanoparticles. The encapsulation of MB in nanoparticles can help to decrease its interaction with the biological milieu and enhance its ability for systemic administration [198].

Theranostics

Multifunctional nanocarriers that can be used for both imaging and therapy of many diseases especially cancer are called theranostics. Theranostics may be conjugated with targeting ligands, imaging agents, and therapeutic agents for both effective imaging and therapy of several diseases especially tumors [46, 199 - 208].

Although it is more common to perform diagnosis and therapy separately in routine applications, targeted theranostics can provide effective diagnosis, imaging, therapy, and follow-up monitoring of tumor response in a single application. Therefore, cancer investigations have transformed to design new and effective nanoparticle-based theranostics for effective cancer diagnosis and treatment [46, 203, 208, 209]. For this purpose, drug delivery systems can carry drugs or therapeutic radionuclides and/or contrast/radiocontrast agents as nanotheranostics by targeting to the target tissue or organ. These nanocarriers exhibit their effect by degrading with lysosomal enzymes in the cells after entering by phagocytosis. In this way, targeted therapy and imaging of cancer can be accomplished.

Drugs, chemotherapeutics, therapeutic radionuclides, or sensitizers which can enhance therapeutic efficacy can be used for tumor therapy. β^- emitting and α emitting radionuclides can also be used for radionuclidic therapy comprising ^{131}I, ^{90}Y, ^{177}Lu, ^{188}Re, ^{201}Ra, ^{211}At, ^{225}Ac, ^{213}Bi, ^{227}Th, *etc* [210 - 212].

As it is widely known, treatment options for glioblastoma are still very limited and ineffective. Doxorubicin hydrochloride (DOX) and SPIO encapsulated, surfactant-coated (Tween 80, Brij-35, Pluronic F68, or Vitamin E-TPGS) polymer poly-Lactic-co-Glycolic Acid (PLGA) nanoparticles were developed for the diagnosis and therapy of glioma. Their diagnostic efficacy was tested by performing MRI relaxivity and therapeutic efficacy in glioma cell lines (U87-MG, 9L/LacZ, and patient derived-neuronal stem cells). Nanoparticles exhibited fine relaxivity and therapeutic efficacy *in vitro* [213].

He *et al.* developed methylene blue (MB) encapsulated bifunctional phosphonate-terminated silica nanoparticles (PSiNPs) for *in vivo* imaging and PDT. Due to the preparation method of MB encapsulated PSiNPs, MB was protected from the leakage through the particles and the reduction by diaphorase. It was reported that 635 nm of light irradiation to MB encapsulated PsiNPs and caused the efficient generation of singlet oxygen and PDT to Hela cells. MB encapsulated PSiNPs were found effective in NIR imaging and PDT as a theranostic approach *in vivo* [214].

The high expression of GPCR neurokinin type 1 receptor (NK-1R) and a modified substance P in glioblastoma may be used for targeting of GBM cells for imaging or therapy. Królicki *et al.* evaluated the therapeutic efficacy of targeted alpha therapy with ^{213}Bi-labeled DOTA-Substance P (^{213}Bi-DOTA-SP) for selective irradiation and tumor cell death. For this purpose, patients were treated with 1–7 doses of ^{213}Bi-DOTA-Substance P in a 2-months interval. To determine the biodistribution by PET/CT, ^{68}Ga-DOTA-SP was co-injected with ^{213}Bi-DOTA-SP. It was observed that the treatment of recurrent GBM with ^{213}Bi-DOTA-SP was a safe and alternative treatment option for recurrent GBM [215]. Therefore, research about nanotheranostics in glioma diagnosis, imaging, and also therapy seems to play a huge role in effective and early personalized therapy in the near future.

CONCLUSION

Due to high heterogeneity and aggressiveness, gliomas have become the subject of numerous research studies. Although MRI is one of the most frequently used methods for the diagnosis and imaging of glioma in routine clinical applications, it is limited in the monitoring of recurrence, therapy response, and pseudoprogression after radiotherapy or combined chemotherapy especially in high-grade gliomas. Hybrid molecular imaging techniques such as PET/CT, SPECT/CT, or PET/MRI can overcome the limitations of single imaging modalities by conjugating functional and anatomical information. They are significant in obtaining accurate, high sensitive, and specific semiquantitative data for glioma imaging. An early and accurate diagnosis can be achieved before the formation of morphological alterations by molecular imaging techniques. For this purpose, radiolabeled nanocarriers have been designed which can participate in tumor cell metabolism in the natural process by targeting tumor metabolism such as glucose, oxygen, and amino acid transport. Cooperation of imaging modalities and nanotechnology with effective, target-specific, novel contrast/radiocontrast and nanotheranostic agents is essential for early diagnosis, accurate imaging, therapy, grading, monitoring of radiotherapy and combined chemotherapy, differentiation of necrosis and inflammation from tumor recurrence and pseudoprogression for glioma.

CONSENT FOR PUBLICATION

Not Applicable.

CONFLICT OF INTEREST

The author confirms that the content of this chapter has no conflict of interest.

ACKNOWLEDGEMENTS

None declared.

REFERENCES

[1]   Wirsching HG, Galanis E, Weller M. Glioblastoma. In: Deisenhammer F, Teunissen CE, Tumani H, Eds. Handbook of Clinical Neurology. 1ˢᵗ ed. New York: Elsevier 2016; pp. 1-446.

[2]   Kılıç T. Available from: http://www.beyincerrahisi.net/beyinomuriliktumorleri/ glioblastoma.html

[3]   Albayrak SB, Beyin Tumoru. Available from: http://www.beyintm.com/ glioblastoma-multiform--gbm.html

[4]   Ozdemir-Kaynak E, Qutub AA, Yesil-Celiktas O. Advances in glioblastoma multiforme treatment: new models for nanoparticle therapy. Front Physiol 2018; 9(1): 170.
[http://dx.doi.org/10.3389/fphys.2018.00170] [PMID: 29615917]

[5]   Kim SS, Harford JB, Pirollo KF, Chang EH. Effective treatment of glioblastoma requires crossing the blood-brain barrier and targeting tumors including cancer stem cells: The promise of nanomedicine. Biochem Biophys Res Commun 2015; 468(3): 485-9.
[http://dx.doi.org/10.1016/j.bbrc.2015.06.137] [PMID: 26116770]

[6]   van Tellingen O, Yetkin-Arik B, de Gooijer MC, Wesseling P, Wurdinger T, de Vries HE. Overcoming the blood-brain tumor barrier for effective glioblastoma treatment. Drug Resist Updat 2015; 19(1): 1-12.
[http://dx.doi.org/10.1016/j.drup.2015.02.002] [PMID: 25791797]

[7]   Yang J, Li Y, Zhang T, Zhang X. Development of bioactive materials for glioblastoma therapy. Bioact Mater 2016; 1(1): 29-38.
[http://dx.doi.org/10.1016/j.bioactmat.2016.03.003] [PMID: 29744393]

[8]   Vigneswaran K, Neill S, Hadjipanayis CG. Beyond the World Health Organization grading of infiltrating gliomas: advances in the molecular genetics of glioma classification. Ann Transl Med 2015; 3(7): 95.
[PMID: 26015937]

[9]   Louis DN, Perry A, Reifenberger G, *et al.* The 2016 World Health Organization classification of tumors of the central nervous system: a summary. Acta Neuropathol 2016; 131(6): 803-20.
[http://dx.doi.org/10.1007/s00401-016-1545-1] [PMID: 27157931]

[10]   Tamimi AF, Juweid M. Epidemiology and outcome of glioblastoma.Glioblastoma. Codon Publications 2017; pp. 143-54.
[http://dx.doi.org/10.15586/codon.glioblastoma.2017.ch8]

[11]   Guilloteau D, Vergote J, Maia S. Importance of radiopharmacy in hospital practice: application to Alzheimer and Parkinson's disease exploration. FABAD J Pharm Sci 2007; 32(1): 41-8.

[12]   Wagner HN, Ed. Principles of nuclear medicine. Philadelphia, USA: W B Saunders Company 1995.

[13]   Boellaard R. Obtaining cardiac images from positron emission tomography, computed tomography, and magnetic resonance imaging: physical principles. Heart Metab 2007; 34(1): 33-7.

[14]   Zimmer L, Rbah L, Giacomelli F, Le Bars D, Renaud B. A reduced extracellular serotonin level increases the 5-HT1A PET ligand 18F-MPPF binding in the rat hippocampus. J Nucl Med 2003; 44(9): 1495-501.
[PMID: 12960198]

[15]   Wen PY, Macdonald DR, Reardon DA, *et al.* Updated response assessment criteria for high-grade gliomas: response assessment in neuro-oncology working group. J Clin Oncol 2010; 28(11): 1963-72.
[http://dx.doi.org/10.1200/JCO.2009.26.3541] [PMID: 20231676]

[16]   Jacobs AH, Kracht LW, Gossmann A, *et al.* Imaging in neurooncology. NeuroRx 2005; 2(2): 333-47.
[http://dx.doi.org/10.1602/neurorx.2.2.333] [PMID: 15897954]

[17]   Götz I, Grosu AL. [18F]FET-PET imaging for treatment and response monitoring of radiation therapy in malignant glioma patients – a review. Front Oncol 2013; 3(1): 104.
[http://dx.doi.org/10.3389/fonc.2013.00104] [PMID: 23630666]

[18]   Iwata Y, Kawamoto M, Yoshizawa Y. Half-life of 68Ga. Int J Appl Radiat Isot 1983; 34(1): 1537-40.
[http://dx.doi.org/10.1016/0020-708X(83)90289-2]

[19]   Velikyan I. 68Ga-Based radiopharmaceuticals: production and application relationship. Molecules 2015; 20(7): 12913-43.
[http://dx.doi.org/10.3390/molecules200712913] [PMID: 26193247]

[20]   Derlon JM, Bourdet C, Bustany P, *et al.* [11C]L-methionine uptake in gliomas. Neurosurgery 1989; 25(5): 720-8.
[http://dx.doi.org/10.1227/00006123-198911000-00006] [PMID: 2586726]

[21]   Heiss P, Mayer S, Herz M, Wester HJ, Schwaiger M, Senekowitsch-Schmidtke R. Investigation of transport mechanism and uptake kinetics of O-(2-[18F]fluoroethyl)-L-tyrosine *in vitro* and *in vivo*. J Nucl Med 1999; 40(8): 1367-73.
[PMID: 10450690]

[22]   Grosu AL, Astner ST, Riedel E, *et al.* An interindividual comparison of O-(2-[18F]fluoroethyl--L-tyrosine (FET)- and L-[methyl-11C]methionine (MET)-PET in patients with brain gliomas and metastases. Int J Radiat Oncol Biol Phys 2011; 81(4): 1049-58.
[http://dx.doi.org/10.1016/j.ijrobp.2010.07.002] [PMID: 21570201]

[23]   Miyagawa T, Oku T, Uehara H, *et al.* "Facilitated" amino acid transport is upregulated in brain tumors. J Cereb Blood Flow Metab 1998; 18(5): 500-9.
[http://dx.doi.org/10.1097/00004647-199805000-00005] [PMID: 9591842]

[24]   Folkman J. Tumor angiogenesis: therapeutic implications. N Engl J Med 1971; 285(21): 1182-6.
[http://dx.doi.org/10.1056/NEJM197111182852108] [PMID: 4938153]

[25]   Hicklin DJ, Ellis LM. Role of the vascular endothelial growth factor pathway in tumor growth and angiogenesis. J Clin Oncol 2005; 23(5): 1011-27.
[http://dx.doi.org/10.1200/JCO.2005.06.081] [PMID: 15585754]

[26]   Louis DN, Ohgaki H, Wiestler OD, *et al.* The 2007 WHO classification of tumours of the central nervous system. Acta Neuropathol 2007; 114(2): 97-109.
[http://dx.doi.org/10.1007/s00401-007-0243-4] [PMID: 17618441]

[27]   Dvorak HF. Vascular permeability factor/vascular endothelial growth factor: a critical cytokine in tumor angiogenesis and a potential target for diagnosis and therapy. J Clin Oncol 2002; 20(21): 4368-80.
[http://dx.doi.org/10.1200/JCO.2002.10.088] [PMID: 12409337]

[28]   Jain RK, Duda DG, Clark JW, Loeffler JS. Lessons from phase III clinical trials on anti-VEGF therapy for cancer. Nat Clin Pract Oncol 2006; 3(1): 24-40.
[http://dx.doi.org/10.1038/ncponc0403] [PMID: 16407877]

[29]   Gil-Gil MJ, Mesia C, Rey M, Bruna J. Bevacizumab for the treatment of glioblastoma. Clin Med Insights Oncol 2013; 7(1): 123-35.
[PMID: 23843722]

[30]   European Medicines Agency.. Avastin (bevacizumab) product page. Available from: http://www.ema.europa.eu/ docs en GB/

[31]   Li Y, Ali S, Clarke J, Cha S. Bevacizumab in Recurrent Glioma: Patterns of Treatment Failure and Implications. Brain Tumor Res Treat 2017; 5(1): 1-9.
[http://dx.doi.org/10.14791/btrt.2017.5.1.1] [PMID: 28516072]

[32]   Clark AS, Deans B, Stevens MF, *et al.* Antitumor imidazotetrazines. 32. Synthesis of novel imidazotetrazinones and related bicyclic heterocycles to probe the mode of action of the antitumor drug temozolomide. J Med Chem 1995; 38(9): 1493-504.
[http://dx.doi.org/10.1021/jm00009a010] [PMID: 7739008]

[33]   Stevens MFG, Hickman JA, Langdon SP, *et al.* Antitumor activity and pharmacokinetics in mice of 8-carbamoyl-3-methyl-imidazo[5,1-d]-1,2,3,5-tetrazin-4(3H)-one (CCRG 81045; M & B 39831), a novel drug with potential as an alternative to dacarbazine. Cancer Res 1987; 47(22): 5846-52.
[PMID: 3664486]

[34]   Friedman HS, Dolan ME, Pegg AE, *et al.* Activity of temozolomide in the treatment of central nervous system tumor xenografts. Cancer Res 1995; 55(13): 2853-7.
[PMID: 7796412]

[35]   Plowman J, Waud WR, Koutsoukos AD, Rubinstein LV, Moore TD, Grever MR. Preclinical antitumor activity of temozolomide in mice: efficacy against human brain tumor xenografts and synergism with 1,3-bis(2-chloroethyl)-1-nitrosourea. Cancer Res 1994; 54(14): 3793-9.
[PMID: 8033099]

[36]   Pera MF, Köberle B, Masters JRW. Exceptional sensitivity of testicular germ cell tumour cell lines to the new anti-cancer agent, temozolomide. Br J Cancer 1995; 71(5): 904-6.
[http://dx.doi.org/10.1038/bjc.1995.176] [PMID: 7734313]

[37]   Carter CA, Waud WR, Plowman J. Responses of human melanoma, ovarian, and colon tumor xenografts in nude mice to oral temozolomide. PAM Assoc Canc Res 1994; 35(1): 297.

[38]   Wedge SR, Porteous JK, Newlands ES. Effect of single and multiple administration of an O6-benzylguanine/temozolomide combination: an evaluation in a human melanoma xenograft model. Cancer Chemother Pharmacol 1997; 40(3): 266-72.
[http://dx.doi.org/10.1007/s002800050657] [PMID: 9219512]

[39]   Patel M, McCully C, Godwin K, Balis F. Plasma and cerebrospinal fluid pharmacokinetics of temozolomide. PAM Assoc Clin Oncol 1995; 14(1): 461.

[40]   Friedman HS, Kerby T, Calvert H. Temozolomide and treatment of malignant glioma. Clin Cancer Res 2000; 6(7): 2585-97.
[PMID: 10914698]

[41]   Xu G, Mahajan S, Roy I, Yong KT. Theranostic quantum dots for crossing blood-brain barrier *in vitro* and providing therapy of HIV-associated encephalopathy. Front Pharmacol 2013; 4(1): 140.
[http://dx.doi.org/10.3389/fphar.2013.00140] [PMID: 24298256]

[42]   Pardridge WM. Drug delivery to the brain. J Cereb Blood Flow Metab 1997; 17(7): 713-31.
[http://dx.doi.org/10.1097/00004647-199707000-00001] [PMID: 9270488]

[43]   Jain RK. Transport of molecules, particles, and cells in solid tumors. Annu Rev Biomed Eng 1999; 1(1): 241-63.
[http://dx.doi.org/10.1146/annurev.bioeng.1.1.241] [PMID: 11701489]

[44]   Fang J, Nakamura H, Maeda H. The EPR effect: Unique features of tumor blood vessels for drug delivery, factors involved, and limitations and augmentation of the effect. Adv Drug Deliv Rev 2011; 63(3): 136-51.
[http://dx.doi.org/10.1016/j.addr.2010.04.009] [PMID: 20441782]

[45]   Greish K. Enhanced permeability and retention (EPR) effect for anticancer nanomedicine drug targeting. Methods Mol Biol 2010; 624(1): 25-37.
[http://dx.doi.org/10.1007/978-1-60761-609-2_3] [PMID: 20217587]

[46]   Bhojani MS, Van Dort M, Rehemtulla A, Ross BD. Targeted imaging and therapy of brain cancer using theranostic nanoparticles. Mol Pharm 2010; 7(6): 1921-9.
[http://dx.doi.org/10.1021/mp100298r] [PMID: 20964352]

[47]   Maeda H, Bharate GY, Daruwalla J. Polymeric drugs for efficient tumor-targeted drug delivery based on EPR-effect. Eur J Pharm Biopharm 2009; 71(3): 409-19.
[http://dx.doi.org/10.1016/j.ejpb.2008.11.010] [PMID: 19070661]

[48]   Gidwani B, Vyas A. A comprehensive review on cyclodextrin-based carriers for delivery of chemotherapeutic cytotoxic anticancer drugs. BioMed Res Int 2015; 2015(1)198268
[http://dx.doi.org/10.1155/2015/198268] [PMID: 26582104]

[49]   Llenas M, Sandoval S, Costa PM, *et al.* Microwave-assisted synthesis of spion-reduced graphene oxide hybrids for magnetic resonance imaging (MRI). Nanomaterials (Basel) 2019; 9(10): 1364.
[http://dx.doi.org/10.3390/nano9101364] [PMID: 31554159]

[50]   Salanci BV. İntrakraniyal tümorlerde moleküler görüntüleme. Türk Radyoloji Seminerleri 2016; 4(1): 59-71.
[http://dx.doi.org/10.5152/trs.2016.341]

[51]   Hottinger AF, Levivier M, Negretti L, Homicsko K, Stupp R. PET imaging in glioma: The neuro-oncologist's expectations. PET Clin 2013; 8(2): 117-28.
[http://dx.doi.org/10.1016/j.cpet.2012.09.006] [PMID: 27157943]

[52]   Santra A, Kumar R, Sharma P, *et al.* F-18 FDG PET-CT in patients with recurrent glioma: comparison with contrast enhanced MRI. Eur J Radiol 2012; 81(3): 508-13.
[http://dx.doi.org/10.1016/j.ejrad.2011.01.080] [PMID: 21353420]

[53]   Kao HW, Chiang SW, Chung HW, Tsai FY, Chen CY. Advanced MR imaging of gliomas: an update. BioMed Res Int 2013; 2013(1)970586
[http://dx.doi.org/10.1155/2013/970586] [PMID: 23862163]

[54]   Noguchi K, Watanabe N, Nagayoshi T, *et al.* Role of diffusion-weighted echo-planar MRI in distinguishing between brain brain abscess and tumour: a preliminary report. Neuroradiology 1999; 41(3): 171-4.
[http://dx.doi.org/10.1007/s002340050726] [PMID: 10206159]

[55]   Stadnik TW, Chaskis C, Michotte A, *et al.* Diffusion-weighted MR imaging of intracerebral masses: comparison with conventional MR imaging and histologic findings. AJNR Am J Neuroradiol 2001; 22(5): 969-76.
[PMID: 11337344]

[56]   Zhang H, Wang T, Zheng Y, Yan C, Gu W, Ye L. Comparative toxicity and contrast enhancing assessments of Gd_2O_3@BSA and MnO_2@BSA nanoparticles for MR imaging of brain glioma. Biochem Biophys Res Commun 2018; 499(3): 488-92.
[http://dx.doi.org/10.1016/j.bbrc.2018.03.175] [PMID: 29580992]

[57]   Morita N, Wang S, Chawla S, Poptani H, Melhem ER. Dynamic susceptibility contrast perfusion weighted imaging in grading of nonenhancing astrocytomas. J Magn Reson Imaging 2010; 32(4): 803-8.
[http://dx.doi.org/10.1002/jmri.22324] [PMID: 20882610]

[58]   Xia D, Davis RL, Crawford JA, Abraham JL. Gadolinium released from MR contrast agents is deposited in brain tumors: *in situ* demonstration using scanning electron microscopy with energy dispersive X-ray spectroscopy. Acta Radiol 2010; 51(10): 1126-36.
[http://dx.doi.org/10.3109/02841851.2010.515614] [PMID: 20868305]

[59]   Kiviniemi A, Gardberg M, Ek P, Frantzén J, Bobacka J, Minn H. Gadolinium retention in gliomas and adjacent normal brain tissue: association with tumor contrast enhancement and linear/macrocyclic agents. Neuroradiology 2019; 61(5): 535-44.
[http://dx.doi.org/10.1007/s00234-019-02172-6] [PMID: 30710184]

[60]   Patil R, Galstyan A, Grodzinski ZB, *et al.* Single- and multi-arm gadolinium MRI contrast agents for targeted imaging of glioblastoma. Int J Nanomedicine 2020; 15(1): 3057-70.
[http://dx.doi.org/10.2147/IJN.S238265] [PMID: 32431501]

[61]   Fonchy E, Lahrech H, François-Joubert A, *et al.* A new gadolinium-based contrast agent for magnetic resonance imaging of brain tumors: kinetic study on a C6 rat glioma model. J Magn Reson Imaging 2001; 14(2): 97-105.
[http://dx.doi.org/10.1002/jmri.1158] [PMID: 11477666]

[62]   He T, Smith N, Saunders D, *et al.* Molecular MRI assessment of vascular endothelial growth factor receptor-2 in rat C6 gliomas. J Cell Mol Med 2010; 1(1): 1582-4934.
[PMID: 20497492]

[63]   Towner RA, Smith N, Asano Y, *et al.* Molecular magnetic resonance imaging approaches used to aid in the understanding of angiogenesis *in vivo*: implications for tissue engineering. Tissue Eng Part A 2010; 16(2): 357-64.
[http://dx.doi.org/10.1089/ten.tea.2009.0233] [PMID: 19663584]

[64]   Towner RA, Smith N, Doblas S, *et al.* *In vivo* detection of c-Met expression in a rat C6 glioma model. J Cell Mol Med 2008; 12(1): 174-86.
[http://dx.doi.org/10.1111/j.1582-4934.2008.00220.x] [PMID: 18194445]

[65]   Towner RA, Smith N, Asano Y, *et al.* Molecular magnetic resonance imaging approaches used to aid in the understanding of the tissue regeneration marker Met *in vivo*: implications for tissue engineering. Tissue Eng Part A 2010; 16(2): 365-71.
[http://dx.doi.org/10.1089/ten.tea.2009.0234] [PMID: 19905873]

[66]   Towner RA, Smith N, Doblas S, *et al.* *In vivo* detection of inducible nitric oxide synthase in rodent gliomas. Free Radic Biol Med 2010; 48(5): 691-703.
[http://dx.doi.org/10.1016/j.freeradbiomed.2009.12.012] [PMID: 20034558]

[67]   Towner RA, He T, Doblas S, Smith N. Assessment of rodent glioma models using magnetic resonance imaging techniques.advances in the biology, imaging and therapies for glioblastoma. USA: IntechOpen 2011; pp. 237-57.

[68]   Kiraz M, Çevik S, Demirel A, Gergin YE, Özdemir Ö. Nanoteknoloji ve Nanonöroşirürji. Türk Nöroşir Derg 2018; 28(3): 264-72.

[69]   Laurent S, Forge D, Port M, *et al.* Magnetic iron oxide nanoparticles: synthesis, stabilization, vectorization, physicochemical characterizations, and biological applications. Chem Rev 2008; 108(6): 2064-110.
[http://dx.doi.org/10.1021/cr068445e] [PMID: 18543879]

[70]   Veiseh O, Gunn JW, Zhang M. Design and fabrication of magnetic nanoparticles for targeted drug delivery and imaging. Adv Drug Deliv Rev 2010; 62(3): 284-304.
[http://dx.doi.org/10.1016/j.addr.2009.11.002] [PMID: 19909778]

[71]   Liu H, Zhang J, Chen X, *et al.* Application of iron oxide nanoparticles in glioma imaging and therapy: from bench to bedside. Nanoscale 2016; 8(15): 7808-26.
[http://dx.doi.org/10.1039/C6NR00147E] [PMID: 27029509]

[72]   Xie H, Zhu Y, Jiang W, *et al.* Lactoferrin-conjugated superparamagnetic iron oxide nanoparticles as a specific MRI contrast agent for detection of brain glioma *in vivo*. Biomaterials 2011; 32(2): 495-502.
[http://dx.doi.org/10.1016/j.biomaterials.2010.09.024] [PMID: 20970851]

[73]   Li W, Szoka FC Jr. Lipid-based nanoparticles for nucleic acid delivery. Pharm Res 2007; 24(3): 438-49.
[http://dx.doi.org/10.1007/s11095-006-9180-5] [PMID: 17252188]

[74]   Giese A, Bjerkvig R, Berens ME, Westphal M. Cost of migration: invasion of malignant gliomas and implications for treatment. J Clin Oncol 2003; 21(8): 1624-36.
[http://dx.doi.org/10.1200/JCO.2003.05.063] [PMID: 12697889]

[75]   Sun C, Veiseh O, Gunn J, *et al. In vivo* MRI detection of gliomas by chlorotoxin-conjugated superparamagnetic nanoprobes. Small 2008; 4(3): 372-9.
[http://dx.doi.org/10.1002/smll.200700784] [PMID: 18232053]

[76]   Reddy GR, Bhojani MS, McConville P, *et al.* Vascular targeted nanoparticles for imaging and treatment of brain tumors. Clin Cancer Res 2006; 12(22): 6677-86.
[http://dx.doi.org/10.1158/1078-0432.CCR-06-0946] [PMID: 17121886]

[77]   Wankhede M, Bouras A, Kaluzova M, Hadjipanayis CG. Magnetic nanoparticles: an emerging technology for malignant brain tumor imaging and therapy. Expert Rev Clin Pharmacol 2012; 5(2): 173-86.
[http://dx.doi.org/10.1586/ecp.12.1] [PMID: 22390560]

[78]   Ancri D, Basset JY. Diagnosis of cerebral metastases by thallium 201. Br J Radiol 1980; 53(629): 443-53.
[http://dx.doi.org/10.1259/0007-1285-53-629-443] [PMID: 7388277]

[79]   Oriuchi N, Tamura M, Shibazaki T, *et al.* Clinical evaluation of thallium-201 SPECT in supratentorial gliomas: relationship to histologic grade, prognosis and proliferative activities. J Nucl Med 1993; 34(12): 2085-9.
[PMID: 8254391]

[80]   Soricelli A, Cuocolo A, Varrone A, *et al.* Technetium-99m-tetrofosmin uptake in brain tumors by SPECT: comparison with thallium-201 imaging. J Nucl Med 1998; 39(5): 802-6.
[PMID: 9591579]

[81]   O'Tuama LA, Treves ST, Larar JN, *et al.* Thallium-201 *versus* technetium-99m-MIBI SPECT in evaluation of childhood brain tumors: a within-subject comparison. J Nucl Med 1993; 34(7): 1045-51.
[PMID: 8315477]

[82]   Soler C, Beauchesne P, Maatougui K, *et al.* Technetium-99m sestamibi brain single-photon emission tomography for detection of recurrent gliomas after radiation therapy. Eur J Nucl Med 1998; 25(12): 1649-57.
[http://dx.doi.org/10.1007/s002590050344] [PMID: 9871097]

[83]   Nishiyama Y, Yamamoto Y, Fukunaga K, Satoh K, Kunishio K, Ohkawa M. Comparison of 99Tcm-MIBI with 201Tl chloride SPET in patients with malignant brain tumours. Nucl Med Commun 2001; 22(6): 631-9.
[http://dx.doi.org/10.1097/00006231-200106000-00005] [PMID: 11403173]

[84]   Biersack HJ, Coenen HH, Stöcklin G, *et al.* Imaging of brain tumors with L-3-[123I]iodo-alha-methyl tyrosine and SPECT. J Nucl Med 1989; 30(1): 110-2.
[PMID: 2783455]

[85]   Kuwert T, Morgenroth C, Woesler B, *et al.* Uptake of iodine-123-alpha-methyl tyrosine by gliomas and non-neoplastic brain lesions. Eur J Nucl Med 1996; 23(10): 1345-53.
[http://dx.doi.org/10.1007/BF01367590] [PMID: 8781139]

[86]   Kuwert T, Woesler B, Morgenroth C, *et al.* Diagnosis of recurrent glioma with SPECT and iodine-123-alpha-methyl tyrosine. J Nucl Med 1998; 39(1): 23-7.
[PMID: 9443732]

[87]   Weber W, Bartenstein P, Gross MW, *et al.* Fluorine-18-FDG PET and iodine-123-IMT SPECT in the evaluation of brain tumors. J Nucl Med 1997; 38(5): 802-8.
[PMID: 9170450]

[88]   Patronas NJ, Di Chiro G, Brooks RA, *et al.* Work in progress: [18F] fluorodeoxyglucose and positron emission tomography in the evaluation of radiation necrosis of the brain. Radiology 1982; 144(4): 885-9.
[http://dx.doi.org/10.1148/radiology.144.4.6981123] [PMID: 6981123]

[89]   Yano H, Shinoda J, Iwama T. Clinical utility of positron emission tomography in patients with

malignant glioma. Neurol Med Chir (Tokyo) 2017; 57(7): 312-20.
[http://dx.doi.org/10.2176/nmc.ra.2016-0312] [PMID: 28458384]

[90]   Verger A, Lange KJ. PET imaging in glioblastoma: Use in clinical practice. In: Vleeschouwer S De, Ed. Glioblastoma. Brisbane (AU): Codon Publications 2017; pp. 154-74.
[http://dx.doi.org/10.15586/codon.glioblastoma.2017.ch9]

[91]   Ocak M. Radiopharmaceuticals for PET. Toraks Cerrahisi Bulteni 2015; 6(1): 154-60.
[http://dx.doi.org/10.5152/tcb.2015.056]

[92]   la Fougère C, Suchorska B, Bartenstein P, Kreth FW, Tonn JC. Molecular imaging of gliomas with PET: opportunities and limitations. Neuro-oncol 2011; 13(8): 806-19.
[http://dx.doi.org/10.1093/neuonc/nor054] [PMID: 21757446]

[93]   Langen KJ, Stoffels G, Filss C, et al. Imaging of amino acid transport in brain tumours: Positron emission tomography with O-(2-[^{18}F]fluoroethyl)-L-tyrosine (FET). Methods 2017; 130(1): 124-34.
[http://dx.doi.org/10.1016/j.ymeth.2017.05.019] [PMID: 28552264]

[94]   Langen KJ, Tonn JC, Weller M, Galldiks N. The role of imaging in the management of progressive glioblastoma. A systematic review and evidencebased clinical practice guideline. J Neurooncol. 2014; 118: pp. 435-60.

[95]   Parent EE, Sharma A, Jain M. Amino Acid PET Imaging of Glioma. Curr Radiol Rep 2019; 7: 14.
[http://dx.doi.org/10.1007/s40134-019-0324-x]

[96]   Kracht LW, Miletic H, Busch S, et al. Delineation of brain tumor extent with [11C]L-methionine positron emission tomography: local comparison with stereotactic histopathology. Clin Cancer Res 2004; 10(21): 7163-70.
[http://dx.doi.org/10.1158/1078-0432.CCR-04-0262] [PMID: 15534088]

[97]   Sharma R, D'Souza M, Jaimini A, et al. A comparison study of (11)C-methionine and (18)F-fluorodeoxyglucose positron emission tomography-computed tomography scans in evaluation of patients with recurrent brain tumors. Indian J Nucl Med 2016; 31(2): 93-102.
[http://dx.doi.org/10.4103/0972-3919.178254] [PMID: 27095856]

[98]   Glaudemans AW, Enting RH, Heesters MA, et al. Value of 11C-methionine PET in imaging brain tumours and metastases. Eur J Nucl Med Mol Imaging 2013; 40(4): 615-35.
[http://dx.doi.org/10.1007/s00259-012-2295-5] [PMID: 23232505]

[99]   Shinozaki N, Uchino Y, Yoshikawa K, et al. Discrimination between low-grade oligodendrogliomas and diffuse astrocytoma with the aid of 11C-methionine positron emission tomography. J Neurosurg 2011; 114(6): 1640-7.
[http://dx.doi.org/10.3171/2010.11.JNS10553] [PMID: 21214332]

[100] Kebir S, Weber M, Lazaridis L, et al. Hybrid ^{11}C-MET PET/MRI combined with machine learning in glioma diagnosis according to the revised glioma WHO classification 2016. Clin Nucl Med 2019; 44(3): 214-20.
[http://dx.doi.org/10.1097/RLU.0000000000002398] [PMID: 30516675]

[101] Takei H, Shinoda J, Ikuta S, et al. Usefulness of positron emission tomography for differentiating gliomas according to the 2016 World Health Organization classification of tumors of the central nervous system. J Neurosurg 2019; 16(1): 1-10.
[http://dx.doi.org/10.3171/2019.5.JNS19780] [PMID: 31419796]

[102] Ozaki T, Kinoshita M, Arita H, et al. Validation of magnetic resonance imaging-based automatic high-grade glioma segmentation accuracy via ^{11}C-methionine positron emission tomography. Oncol Lett 2019; 18(4): 4074-81.
[http://dx.doi.org/10.3892/ol.2019.10734] [PMID: 31516607]

[103] Michaud L, Beattie BJ, Akhurst T, et al. ^{18}F-Fluciclovine (^{18}F-FACBC) PET imaging of recurrent brain tumors. Eur J Nucl Med Mol Imaging 2019; 1(1): 1-15.
[PMID: 31418054]

[104]   Kato T, Shinoda J, Nakayama N, *et al.* Metabolic assessment of gliomas using 11C-methionine, [18F] fluorodeoxyglucose, and 11C-choline positron-emission tomography. AJNR Am J Neuroradiol 2008; 29(6): 1176-82.
[http://dx.doi.org/10.3174/ajnr.A1008] [PMID: 18388218]

[105]   Pirotte B, Goldman S, Dewitte O, *et al.* Integrated positron emission tomography and magnetic resonance imaging-guided resection of brain tumors: a report of 103 consecutive procedures. J Neurosurg 2006; 104(2): 238-53.
[http://dx.doi.org/10.3171/jns.2006.104.2.238] [PMID: 16509498]

[106]   Gumprecht H, Grosu AL, Souvatsoglou M, Dzewas B, Weber WA, Lumenta CB. 11C-Methionine positron emission tomography for preoperative evaluation of suggestive low-grade gliomas. Zentralbl Neurochir 2007; 68(1): 19-23.
[http://dx.doi.org/10.1055/s-2007-970601] [PMID: 17487804]

[107]   Lee IH, Piert M, Gomez-Hassan D, *et al.* Association of 11C-methionine PET uptake with site of failure after concurrent temozolomide and radiation for primary glioblastoma multiforme. Int J Radiat Oncol Biol Phys 2009; 73(2): 479-85.
[http://dx.doi.org/10.1016/j.ijrobp.2008.04.050] [PMID: 18834673]

[108]   Ono T, Sasajima T, Doi Y, *et al.* Amino acid PET tracers are reliable markers of treatment responses to single-agent or combination therapies including temozolomide, interferon-β, and/or bevacizumab for glioblastoma. Nucl Med Biol 2015; 42(7): 598-607.
[http://dx.doi.org/10.1016/j.nucmedbio.2015.01.008] [PMID: 25892210]

[109]   Hamacher K, Coenen HH. Efficient routine production of the 18F-labelled amino acid O-2-18F fluoroethyl-L-tyrosine. Appl Radiat Isot 2002; 57(6): 853-6.
[http://dx.doi.org/10.1016/S0969-8043(02)00225-7] [PMID: 12406628]

[110]   Siddiq IS, Atwa ST, Shama SA, Eltaoudy MH, Omar WM. Radiosynthesis and modified quality control of O-(2-[^{18}F]fluoroethyl)-L-tyrosine ([^{18}F]FET) for brain tumor imaging. Appl Radiat Isot 2018; 133(1): 38-44.
[http://dx.doi.org/10.1016/j.apradiso.2017.12.011] [PMID: 29275040]

[111]   Moulin-Romsée G, D'Hondt E, de Groot T, *et al.* Non-invasive grading of brain tumours using dynamic amino acid PET imaging: does it work for 11C-methionine? Eur J Nucl Med Mol Imaging 2007; 34(12): 2082-7.
[http://dx.doi.org/10.1007/s00259-007-0557-4] [PMID: 17763978]

[112]   Gross MW, Weber WA, Feldmann HJ, Bartenstein P, Schwaiger M, Molls M. The value of F-1- -fluorodeoxyglucose PET for the 3-D radiation treatment planning of malignant gliomas. Int J Radiat Oncol Biol Phys 1998; 41(5): 989-95.
[http://dx.doi.org/10.1016/S0360-3016(98)00183-7] [PMID: 9719107]

[113]   Weber DC, Zilli T, Buchegger F, *et al.* [(18)F]Fluoroethyltyrosine- positron emission tomography-guided radiotherapy for high-grade glioma. Radiat Oncol 2008; 3(1): 44.
[http://dx.doi.org/10.1186/1748-717X-3-44] [PMID: 19108742]

[114]   Niyazi M, Geisler J, Siefert A, *et al.* FET-PET for malignant glioma treatment planning. Radiother Oncol 2011; 99(1): 44-8.
[http://dx.doi.org/10.1016/j.radonc.2011.03.001] [PMID: 21458093]

[115]   Piroth MD, Pinkawa M, Holy R, *et al.* Prognostic value of early [^{18}F]fluoroethyltyrosine positron emission tomography after radiochemotherapy in glioblastoma multiforme. Int J Radiat Oncol Biol Phys 2011; 80(1): 176-84.
[http://dx.doi.org/10.1016/j.ijrobp.2010.01.055] [PMID: 20646863]

[116]   Nariai T, Tanaka Y, Wakimoto H, *et al.* Usefulness of L-[methyl-^{11}C] methionine-positron emission tomography as a biological monitoring tool in the treatment of glioma. J Neurosurg 2005; 103(3): 498-507.
[http://dx.doi.org/10.3171/jns.2005.103.3.0498] [PMID: 16235683]

[117]   Wester HJ, Herz M, Weber W, *et al.* Synthesis and radiopharmacology of for tumor imaging. J Nucl Med 1998; 40(1): 205-12.
[PMID: 9935078]

[118]   Kaim AH, Weber B, Kurrer MO, *et al.* (18)F-FDG and (18)F-FET uptake in experimental soft tissue infection. Eur J Nucl Med Mol Imaging 2002; 29(5): 648-54.
[http://dx.doi.org/10.1007/s00259-002-0780-y] [PMID: 11976803]

[119]   Rau FC, Weber WA, Wester HJ, *et al.* O-(2-[(18)F]Fluoroethyl)- L-tyrosine (FET): a tracer for differentiation of tumour from inflammation in murine lymph nodes. Eur J Nucl Med Mol Imaging 2002; 29(8): 1039-46.
[http://dx.doi.org/10.1007/s00259-002-0821-6] [PMID: 12173018]

[120]   Rapp M, Heinzel A, Galldiks N, *et al.* Diagnostic performance of 18F-FET PET in newly diagnosed cerebral lesions suggestive of glioma. J Nucl Med 2013; 54(2): 229-35.
[http://dx.doi.org/10.2967/jnumed.112.109603] [PMID: 23232275]

[121]   Floeth FW, Pauleit D, Sabel M, *et al.* 18F-FET PET differentiation of ring-enhancing brain lesions. J Nucl Med 2006; 47(5): 776-82.
[PMID: 16644747]

[122]   Galldiks N, Langen KJ, Pope WB. From the clinician's point of view - What is the status quo of positron emission tomography in patients with brain tumors? Neuro-oncol 2015; 17(11): 1434-44.
[http://dx.doi.org/10.1093/neuonc/nov118] [PMID: 26130743]

[123]   Calcagni ML, Galli G, Giordano A, *et al.* Dynamic O-(2-[18F]fluoroethyl)-L-tyrosine (F-18 FET) PET for glioma grading: assessment of individual probability of malignancy. Clin Nucl Med 2011; 36(10): 841-7.
[http://dx.doi.org/10.1097/RLU.0b013e3182291b40] [PMID: 21892031]

[124]   Kratochwil C, Combs SE, Leotta K, *et al.* Intra-individual comparison of ^{1}☐F-FET and ^{1}☐F-DOPA in PET imaging of recurrent brain tumors. Neuro-oncol 2014; 16(3): 434-40.
[http://dx.doi.org/10.1093/neuonc/not199] [PMID: 24305717]

[125]   Dunet V, Rossier C, Buck A, Stupp R, Prior JO. Performance of 18F-fluoro-ethyl-tyrosine (18F-FET) PET for the differential diagnosis of primary brain tumor: a systematic review and Metaanalysis. J Nucl Med 2012; 53(2): 207-14.
[http://dx.doi.org/10.2967/jnumed.111.096859] [PMID: 22302961]

[126]   Hutterer M, Nowosielski M, Putzer D, *et al.* [18F]-fluoro-ethyl-L-tyrosine PET: a valuable diagnostic tool in neuro-oncology, but not all that glitters is glioma. Neuro-oncol 2013; 15(3): 341-51.
[http://dx.doi.org/10.1093/neuonc/nos300] [PMID: 23335162]

[127]   Stockhammer F, Plotkin M, Amthauer H, van Landeghem FK, Woiciechowsky C. Correlation of F-1--fluoro-ethyl-tyrosin uptake with vascular and cell density in non-contrast-enhancing gliomas. J Neurooncol 2008; 88(2): 205-10.
[http://dx.doi.org/10.1007/s11060-008-9551-3] [PMID: 18317691]

[128]   Collet S, Valable S, Constans JM, *et al.* [(18)F]-fluoro-L-thymidine PET and advanced MRI for preoperative grading of gliomas. Neuroimage Clin 2015; 8(1): 448-54.
[http://dx.doi.org/10.1016/j.nicl.2015.05.012] [PMID: 26106569]

[129]   Stegmayr C, Oliveira D, Niemietz N, *et al.* Influence of bevacizumab on blood-brain barrier permeability and O -(2- 18 F-Fluoroethyl)-l-tyrosine uptake in rat gliomas. J Nucl Med 2017; 58(5): 700-5.
[http://dx.doi.org/10.2967/jnumed.116.187047] [PMID: 28153956]

[130]   Jansen NL, Suchorska B, Wenter V, *et al.* Dynamic 18F-FET PET in newly diagnosed astrocytic low-grade glioma identifies high-risk patients. J Nucl Med 2014; 55(2): 198-203.
[http://dx.doi.org/10.2967/jnumed.113.122333] [PMID: 24379223]

[131]   Galldiks N, Dunkl V, Stoffels G, *et al.* Diagnosis of pseudoprogression in patients with glioblastoma

using O-(2-[18F]fluoroethyl)-L-tyrosine PET. Eur J Nucl Med Mol Imaging 2015; 42(5): 685-95.
[http://dx.doi.org/10.1007/s00259-014-2959-4] [PMID: 25411133]

[132] Pollack IF, Jakacki RI. Childhood brain tumors: epidemiology, current management and future directions. Nat Rev Neurol 2011; 7(9): 495-506.
[http://dx.doi.org/10.1038/nrneurol.2011.110] [PMID: 21788981]

[133] Dunkl V, Cleff C, Stoffels G, *et al.* The usefulness of dynamic O-(2-18F-fluoroethyl)-L-tyrosine PET in the clinical evaluation of brain tumors in children and adolescents. J Nucl Med 2015; 56(1): 88-92.
[http://dx.doi.org/10.2967/jnumed.114.148734] [PMID: 25525183]

[134] Nedergaard MK, Kristoffersen K, Michaelsen SR, *et al.* The use of longitudinal 18F-FET MicroPET imaging to evaluate response to irinotecan in orthotopic human glioblastoma multiforme xenografts. PLoS One 2014; 9(2)e100009
[http://dx.doi.org/10.1371/journal.pone.0100009] [PMID: 24918622]

[135] Lapa C, Linsenmann T, Monoranu CM, *et al.* Comparison of the amino acid tracers 18F-FET and 18F-DOPA in high-grade glioma patients. J Nucl Med 2014; 55(10): 1611-6.
[http://dx.doi.org/10.2967/jnumed.114.140608] [PMID: 25125481]

[136] Bell C, Dowson N, Puttick S, *et al.* Increasing feasibility and utility of (18)F-FDOPA PET for the management of glioma. Nucl Med Biol 2015; 42(10): 788-95.
[http://dx.doi.org/10.1016/j.nucmedbio.2015.06.001] [PMID: 26162582]

[137] Karunanithi S, Sharma P, Kumar A, *et al.* Comparative diagnostic accuracy of contrast-enhanced MRI and (18)F-FDOPA PET-CT in recurrent glioma. Eur Radiol 2013; 23(9): 2628-35.
[http://dx.doi.org/10.1007/s00330-013-2838-6] [PMID: 23624623]

[138] Ledezma CJ, Chen W, Sai V, *et al.* 18F-FDOPA PET/MRI fusion in patients with primary/recurrent gliomas: initial experience. Eur J Radiol 2009; 71(2): 242-8.
[http://dx.doi.org/10.1016/j.ejrad.2008.04.018] [PMID: 18511228]

[139] Chiaravalloti A, Fiorentini A, Villani V, *et al.* Factors affecting ¹ F FDOPA standardized uptake value in patients with primary brain tumors after treatment. Nucl Med Biol 2015; 42(4): 355-9.
[http://dx.doi.org/10.1016/j.nucmedbio.2015.01.002] [PMID: 25624151]

[140] Ginet M, Zaragori T, Marie PY, *et al.* Integration of dynamic parameters in the analysis of 18F-FDopa PET imaging improves the prediction of molecular features of gliomas. Eur J Nucl Med Mol Imaging 2019; 1(1): 1-10.
[http://dx.doi.org/10.1007/s00259-019-04509-y] [PMID: 31529264]

[141] Fernandez P, Zanotti-Fregonara P, Eimer S, *et al.* Combining 3'-Deoxy-3'-[18F] fluorothymidine and MRI increases the sensitivity of glioma volume detection. Nucl Med Commun 2019; 40(10): 1066-71.
[http://dx.doi.org/10.1097/MNM.0000000000001056] [PMID: 31469809]

[142] Chen W, Cloughesy T, Kamdar N, *et al.* Imaging proliferation in brain tumors with 18F-FLT PET: comparison with 18F-FDG. J Nucl Med 2005; 46(6): 945-52.
[PMID: 15937304]

[143] Corroyer-Dulmont A, Pérès EA, Gérault AN, *et al.* Multimodal imaging based on MRI and PET reveals [(18)F]FLT PET as a specific and early indicator of treatment efficacy in a preclinical model of recurrent glioblastoma. Eur J Nucl Med Mol Imaging 2016; 43(4): 682-94.
[http://dx.doi.org/10.1007/s00259-015-3225-0] [PMID: 26537287]

[144] Shimizu Y, Kudo K, Kameda H, *et al.* Prediction of hypoxia in brain tumors using a multivariate model built from MR imaging and ¹⁸F-Fluorodeoxyglucose accumulation data. Magn Reson Med Sci 2019; 1(1): 1-8.
[PMID: 31611541]

[145] Cher LM, Murone C, Lawrentschuk N, *et al.* Correlation of hypoxic cell fraction and angiogenesis with glucose metabolic rate in gliomas using 18F-fluoromisonidazole, 18F-FDG PET, and immunohistochemical studies. J Nucl Med 2006; 47(3): 410-8.

[PMID: 16513609]

[146] Valk PE, Mathis CA, Prados MD, Gilbert JC, Budinger TF. Hypoxia in human gliomas: demonstration by PET with fluorine-18-fluoromisonidazole. J Nucl Med 1992; 33(12): 2133-7.
[PMID: 1334136]

[147] Bénard F, Romsa J, Hustinx R. Imaging gliomas with positron emission tomography and single-photon emission computed tomography. Semin Nucl Med 2003; 33(2): 148-62.
[http://dx.doi.org/10.1053/snuc.2003.127304] [PMID: 12756647]

[148] Güç D. Adezyon moleküller. ANKEM Derg 2004; 18(2): 158-63.

[149] Chen X, Park R, Shahinian AH, et al. 18F-labeled RGD peptide: initial evaluation for imaging brain tumor angiogenesis. Nucl Med Biol 2004; 31(2): 179-89.
[http://dx.doi.org/10.1016/j.nucmedbio.2003.10.002] [PMID: 15013483]

[150] Gallium 68Ga-labeled BNOTA-PRGD2. NCI Drug Dictionary, National Cancer Institute.. Available from: https://www.cancer.gov/ publications/ dictionaries/cancer-drug?cdrid=725242

[151] Mühlhausen U, Komljenovic D, Bretschi M, et al. A novel PET tracer for the imaging of αvβ3 and αvβ5 integrins in experimental breast cancer bone metastases. Contrast Media Mol Imaging 2011; 6(6): 413-20.
[http://dx.doi.org/10.1002/cmmi.435] [PMID: 22162137]

[152] Li D, Zhao X, Zhang L, et al. (68)Ga-PRGD2 PET/CT in the evaluation of Glioma: a prospective study. Mol Pharm 2014; 11(11): 3923-9.
[http://dx.doi.org/10.1021/mp5003224] [PMID: 25093246]

[153] Notni J, Steiger K, Hoffmann F, et al. Variation of specific activities of 68Ga-Aquibeprin and 68Ga-Avebetrin enables Selective PET imaging of different expression levels of integrins a5b1 and avb3. J Nucl Med 2016; 57(10): 1618-24.
[http://dx.doi.org/10.2967/jnumed.116.173948] [PMID: 27151985]

[154] Haubner R, Kuhnast B, Mang C, et al. [18F]Galacto-RGD: synthesis, radiolabeling, metabolic stability, and radiation dose estimates. Bioconjug Chem 2004; 15(1): 61-9.
[http://dx.doi.org/10.1021/bc034170n] [PMID: 14733584]

[155] Schnell O, Krebs B, Carlsen J, et al. Imaging of integrin alpha(v)beta(3) expression in patients with malignant glioma by [18F] Galacto-RGD positron emission tomography. Neuro-oncol 2009; 11(6): 861-70.
[http://dx.doi.org/10.1215/15228517-2009-024] [PMID: 19401596]

[156] Ecevit H, Motor S, İzmirli M. Genden tedaviye yeni yaklaşımlar: kodlanmayan nükleik asitler. Mustafa Kemal Üniversitesi Tıp Dergisi 2013; 13(4): 26-34.

[157] Tekintaş Y, Demir-Dora D, Hoşgör-Limoncu M. Antisens oligonükleotitler ve antibakteriyel kullanımları. Türk Mikrobiyol Cemiy Derg 2016; 46(2): 51-7.

[158] Tavitian B. In vivo antisense imaging. Q J Nucl Med 2000; 44(3): 236-55.
[PMID: 11105588]

[159] Lendvai G, Estrada S, Bergström M. Radiolabelled oligonucleotides for imaging of gene expression with PET. Curr Med Chem 2009; 16(33): 4445-61.
[http://dx.doi.org/10.2174/092986709789712844] [PMID: 19835563]

[160] Hnatowich DJ, Winnard P, Virzi F, et al. Technetium-99m labeling of DNA oligonucleotides. J Nucl Med 1999; 36(12): 2306-14.

[161] Dewanjee MK, Haider N, Narula J. Imaging with radiolabeled antisense oligonucleotides for the detection of intracellular messenger RNA and cardiovascular disease. J Nucl Cardiol 1999; 6(3): 345-56.
[http://dx.doi.org/10.1016/S1071-3581(99)90047-8] [PMID: 10385190]

[162] Fujibayashi Y, Yoshimi E, Waki A, et al. A novel ^{111}In-labeled antisense DNA probe with multi-

chelating sites (MCS-probe) showing high specific radioactivity and labeling efficiency. Nucl Med Biol 1999; 26(1): 17-21.
[http://dx.doi.org/10.1016/S0969-8051(98)00058-4] [PMID: 10096496]

[163]   Dewanjee MK, Ghafouripour AK, Werner RK, Serafini AN, Sfakianakis GN. Development of sensitive radioiodinated anti-sense oligonucleotide probes by conjugation technique. Bioconjug Chem 1991; 2(4): 195-200.
[http://dx.doi.org/10.1021/bc00010a001] [PMID: 1772900]

[164]   Kühnast B, Dollé F, Terrazzino S, *et al.* General method to label antisense oligonucleotides with radioactive halogens for pharmacological and imaging studies. Bioconjug Chem 2000; 11(5): 627-36.
[http://dx.doi.org/10.1021/bc990183i] [PMID: 10995205]

[165]   Visser G, Vos M, Davenport R, Pike V, Medema J, Vaalburg W. Development of labelled antisense deoxyoligonucleotides (ODNs) for use in PET. Synthesis of the [^{11}C]-labelled dinucleotide [^{11}C]-thymidylyl (3′–5′) thymidine. J Labelled Comp Radiopharm 1995; 37(1): 341-3.

[166]   Kobori N, Imahori Y, Mineura K, Ueda S, Fujii R. Visualization of mRNA expression in CNS using ^{11}C-labeled phosphorothioate oligodeoxynucleotide. Neuroreport 1999; 10(14): 2971-4.
[http://dx.doi.org/10.1097/00001756-199909290-00018] [PMID: 10549807]

[167]   Roivainen A, Tolvanen T, Salomäki S, *et al.* ^{68}Ga-labeled oligonucleotides for *in vivo* imaging with PET. J Nucl Med 2004; 45(2): 347-55.
[PMID: 14960659]

[168]   Kshirsagar NA. Drug delivery systems. Indian J Pharmacol 2000; 32(1): 54-61.

[169]   Jain KK, Ed. Methods in molecular biology-drug delivery systems. USA: Humana Press, Springer 2008.
[http://dx.doi.org/10.1007/978-1-59745-210-6]

[170]   Silindir M, Erdoğan S, Özer AY, Maia S. Liposomes and their applications in molecular imaging. J Drug Target 2012; 20(5): 401-15.
[http://dx.doi.org/10.3109/1061186X.2012.685477] [PMID: 22553977]

[171]   Moghimi SM, Hunter AC. Poloxamers and poloxamines in nanoparticle engineering and experimental medicine. Trends Biotechnol 2000; 18(10): 412-20.
[http://dx.doi.org/10.1016/S0167-7799(00)01485-2] [PMID: 10998507]

[172]   Park EK, Lee SB, Lee YM. Preparation and characterization of methoxy poly(ethylene glycol)/poly(epsilon-caprolactone) amphiphilic block copolymeric nanospheres for tumor-specific folate-mediated targeting of anticancer drugs. Biomaterials 2005; 26(9): 1053-61.
[http://dx.doi.org/10.1016/j.biomaterials.2004.04.008] [PMID: 15369694]

[173]   Piktel E, Niemirowicz K, Wątek M, Wollny T, Deptuła P, Bucki R. Recent insights in nanotechnology-based drugs and formulations designed for effective anti-cancer therapy. J Nanobiotechnology 2016; 14(1): 39.
[http://dx.doi.org/10.1186/s12951-016-0193-x] [PMID: 27229857]

[174]   Ahuja V. Nanoparticle drug delivery for cancer therapy: an update. SF Drug Deliv Res J 2017; 1(1): 2.

[175]   Farokhzad OC, Jon S, Khademhosseini A, Tran TN, Lavan DA, Langer R. Nanoparticle-aptamer bioconjugates: a new approach for targeting prostate cancer cells. Cancer Res 2004; 64(21): 7668-72.
[http://dx.doi.org/10.1158/0008-5472.CAN-04-2550] [PMID: 15520166]

[176]   Gref R, Minamitake Y, Peracchia MT, Trubetskoy V, Torchilin V, Langer R. Biodegradable long-circulating polymeric nanospheres. Science 1994; 263(5153): 1600-3.
[http://dx.doi.org/10.1126/science.8128245] [PMID: 8128245]

[177]   Chari RV. Targeted delivery of chemotherapeutics: tumor-activated prodrug therapy. Adv Drug Deliv Rev 1998; 31(1-2): 89-104.
[http://dx.doi.org/10.1016/S0169-409X(97)00095-1] [PMID: 10837619]

[178] Mansour AM, Drevs J, Esser N, *et al.* A new approach for the treatment of malignant melanoma: enhanced antitumor efficacy of an albumin-binding doxorubicin prodrug that is cleaved by matrix metalloproteinase 2. Cancer Res 2003; 63(14): 4062-6.
[PMID: 12874007]

[179] Guo X, Szoka FC Jr. Chemical approaches to triggerable lipid vesicles for drug and gene delivery. Acc Chem Res 2003; 36(5): 335-41.
[http://dx.doi.org/10.1021/ar9703241] [PMID: 12755643]

[180] Arora D, Jaglan S. Nanocarriers based delivery of nutraceuticals for cancer prevention and treatment: A review of recent research developments. Trends Food Sci Technol 2016; 54(1): 114-26.
[http://dx.doi.org/10.1016/j.tifs.2016.06.003]

[181] Wu W, Zhong S, Gong Y, *et al.* A new molecular probe: An NRP-1 targeting probe for the grading diagnosis of glioma in nude mice. Neurosci Lett 2019; •••: xxx. [xxxx]. [, xxxx.].
[PMID: 31705924]

[182] Kiessling F, Huppert J, Zhang C, *et al.* RGD-labeled USPIO inhibits adhesion and endocytotic activity of α v β3-integrin-expressing glioma cells and only accumulates in the vascular tumor compartment. Radiology 2009; 253(2): 462-9.
[http://dx.doi.org/10.1148/radiol.2532081815] [PMID: 19789239]

[183] Yang L, Shao B, Zhang X, Cheng Q, Lin T, Liu E. Multifunctional upconversion nanoparticles for targeted dual-modal imaging in rat glioma xenograft. J Biomater Appl 2016; 31(3): 400-10.

[184] Shevtsov M, Nikolaev B, Marchenko Y, *et al.* Targeting experimental orthotopic glioblastoma with chitosan-based superparamagnetic iron oxide nanoparticles (CS-DX-SPIONs). Int J Nanomedicine 2018; 13(1): 1471-82.
[http://dx.doi.org/10.2147/IJN.S152461] [PMID: 29559776]

[185] Mamani JB, Malheiros JM, Cardoso EF, Tannús A, Silveira PH, Gamarra LF. *In vivo* magnetic resonance imaging tracking of C6 glioma cells labeled with superparamagnetic iron oxide nanoparticles. Einstein (Sao Paulo) 2012; 10(2): 164-70.
[http://dx.doi.org/10.1590/S1679-45082012000200009] [PMID: 23052451]

[186] Moffat BA, Reddy GR, McConville P, *et al.* A novel polyacrylamide magnetic nanoparticle contrast agent for molecular imaging using MRI. Mol Imaging 2003; 2(4): 324-32.
[http://dx.doi.org/10.1162/153535003322750664] [PMID: 14717331]

[187] Tréhin R, Figueiredo JL, Pittet MJ, Weissleder R, Josephson L, Mahmood U. Fluorescent nanoparticle uptake for brain tumor visualization. Neoplasia 2006; 8(4): 302-11.
[http://dx.doi.org/10.1593/neo.05751] [PMID: 16756722]

[188] Helbok A, Decristoforo C, Dobrozemsky G, *et al.* Radiolabeling of lipid-based nanoparticles for diagnostics and therapeutic applications: a comparison using different radiometals. J Liposome Res 2010; 20(3): 219-27.
[http://dx.doi.org/10.3109/08982100903311812] [PMID: 19863193]

[189] Bouziotis P, Stellas D, Thomas E, *et al.* 68Ga-radiolabeled AGuIX nanoparticles as dual-modality imaging agents for PET/MRI-guided radiation therapy. Nanomedicine (Lond) 2017; 12(13): 1561-74.
[http://dx.doi.org/10.2217/nnm-2017-0032] [PMID: 28621567]

[190] Miladi I, Duc GL, Kryza D, *et al.* Biodistribution of ultra small gadolinium-based nanoparticles as theranostic agent: application to brain tumors. J Biomater Appl 2013; 28(3): 385-94.
[http://dx.doi.org/10.1177/0885328212454315] [PMID: 22832216]

[191] Nigam S, McCarl L, Kumar R, *et al.* Preclinical immunoPET Imaging of glioblastoma-infiltrating myeloid cells using Zirconium-89 labeled anti-CD11b antibody. Mol Imaging Biol 2019; 1(1): 1-10.
[PMID: 29516387]

[192] Li S, Johnson J, Peck A, Xie Q. Near infrared fluorescent imaging of brain tumor with IR780 dye incorporated phospholipid nanoparticles. J Transl Med 2017; 15(1): 18.

[http://dx.doi.org/10.1186/s12967-016-1115-2] [PMID: 28114956]

[193] Zhou H, Luby-Phelps K, Mickey BE, Habib AA, Mason RP, Zhao D. Dynamic near-infrared optical imaging of 2-deoxyglucose uptake by intracranial glioma of athymic mice. PLoS One 2009; 4(11)e8051
[http://dx.doi.org/10.1371/journal.pone.0008051] [PMID: 19956682]

[194] Zheng X, Xing D, Zhou F, Wu B, Chen WR. Indocyanine green-containing nanostructure as near infrared dual-functional targeting probes for optical imaging and photothermal therapy. Mol Pharm 2011; 8(2): 447-56.
[http://dx.doi.org/10.1021/mp100301t] [PMID: 21197955]

[195] Veiseh O, Sun C, Gunn J, *et al.* Optical and MRI multifunctional nanoprobe for targeting gliomas. Nano Lett 2005; 5(6): 1003-8.
[http://dx.doi.org/10.1021/nl0502569] [PMID: 15943433]

[196] Zhang L, Zhao D. Liposomal encapsulation enhances *in vivo* near infrared imaging of exposed phosphatidylserine in a mouse glioma model. Molecules 2013; 18(12): 14613-28.
[http://dx.doi.org/10.3390/molecules181214613] [PMID: 24287994]

[197] Benachour H, Sève A, Bastogne T, *et al.* Multifunctional Peptide-conjugated hybrid silica nanoparticles for photodynamic therapy and MRI. Theranostics 2012; 2(9): 889-904.
[http://dx.doi.org/10.7150/thno.4754] [PMID: 23082101]

[198] Tang W, Xu H, Kopelman R, Philbert MA. Photodynamic characterization and *in vitro* application of methylene blue-containing nanoparticle platforms. Photochem Photobiol 2005; 81(2): 242-9.
[http://dx.doi.org/10.1562/2004-05-24-RA-176.1] [PMID: 15595888]

[199] Liong M, Lu J, Kovochich M, *et al.* Multifunctional inorganic nanoparticles for imaging, targeting, and drug delivery. ACS Nano 2008; 2(5): 889-96.
[http://dx.doi.org/10.1021/nn800072t] [PMID: 19206485]

[200] Medarova Z, Kumar M, Ng SW, *et al.* Multifunctional magnetic nanocarriers for image-tagged SiRNA delivery to intact pancreatic islets. Transplantation 2008; 86(9): 1170-7.
[http://dx.doi.org/10.1097/TP.0b013e31818a81b2] [PMID: 19005396]

[201] Kumar A, Jena PK, Behera S, Lockey RF, Mohapatra S, Mohapatra S. Multifunctional magnetic nanoparticles for targeted delivery. Nanomedicine (Lond) 2010; 6(1): 64-9.
[http://dx.doi.org/10.1016/j.nano.2009.04.002] [PMID: 19446653]

[202] McCarthy JR, Weissleder R. Multifunctional magnetic nanoparticles for targeted imaging and therapy. Adv Drug Deliv Rev 2008; 60(11): 1241-51.
[http://dx.doi.org/10.1016/j.addr.2008.03.014] [PMID: 18508157]

[203] Blanco E, Kessinger CW, Sumer BD, Gao J. Multifunctional micellar nanomedicine for cancer therapy. Exp Biol Med (Maywood) 2009; 234(2): 123-31.
[http://dx.doi.org/10.3181/0808-MR-250] [PMID: 19064945]

[204] Guo R, Zhang L, Qian H, Li R, Jiang X, Liu B. Multifunctional nanocarriers for cell imaging, drug delivery, and near-IR photothermal therapy. Langmuir 2010; 26(8): 5428-34.
[http://dx.doi.org/10.1021/la903893n] [PMID: 20095619]

[205] Bhaskar S, Tian F, Stoeger T, *et al.* Multifunctional Nanocarriers for diagnostics, drug delivery and targeted treatment across blood-brain barrier: perspectives on tracking and neuroimaging. Part Fibre Toxicol 2010; 7(3): 3.
[http://dx.doi.org/10.1186/1743-8977-7-3] [PMID: 20199661]

[206] Gindy ME, Prud'homme RK. Multifunctional nanoparticles for imaging, delivery and targeting in cancer therapy. Expert Opin Drug Deliv 2009; 6(8): 865-78.
[http://dx.doi.org/10.1517/17425240902932908] [PMID: 19637974]

[207] Masotti A. Multifuntional nanoparticles: preparation and applications in biomedicine and in non-invasive bioimaging. Recent Pat Nanotechnol 2010; 4(1): 53-62.

[http://dx.doi.org/10.2174/187221010790712093] [PMID: 20214655]

[208]   Pan D, Lanza GM, Wickline SA, Caruthers SD. Nanomedicine: perspective and promises with ligand-directed molecular imaging. Eur J Radiol 2009; 70(2): 274-85.
[http://dx.doi.org/10.1016/j.ejrad.2009.01.042] [PMID: 19268515]

[209]   Chen W, Bardhan R, Bartels M, *et al.* A molecularly targeted theranostic probe for ovarian cancer. Mol Cancer Ther 2010; 9(4): 1028-38.
[http://dx.doi.org/10.1158/1535-7163.MCT-09-0829] [PMID: 20371708]

[210]   Allard E, Hindre F, Passirani C, *et al.* [188]Re-loaded lipid nanocapsules as a promising radiopharmaceutical carrier for internal radiotherapy of malignant gliomas. Eur J Nucl Med Mol Imaging 2008; 35(10): 1838-46.
[http://dx.doi.org/10.1007/s00259-008-0735-z] [PMID: 18465130]

[211]   Caffo M, Cardali S, Fazzari E, Barresi V, Caruso G. Nanoparticles drug-delivery systems and antiangiogenic approaches in the treatment of gliomas. Glioma 2018; 1(6): 183-8.
[http://dx.doi.org/10.4103/glioma.glioma_43_18]

[212]   Vural G, Özer AY. Drug delivery systems and theranostic use in nuclear medicine. Nucl Med Seminar 2015; 2(1): 109-9.

[213]   Luque-Michel E, Sebastian V, Larrea A, Marquina C, Blanco-Prieto MJ. Co-encapsulation of superparamagnetic nanoparticles and doxorubicin in PLGA nanocarriers: Development, characterization and *in vitro* antitumor efficacy in glioma cells. Eur J Pharm Biopharm 2019; 145(1): 65-75.
[http://dx.doi.org/10.1016/j.ejpb.2019.10.004] [PMID: 31628997]

[214]   He X, Wu X, Wang K, Shi B, Hai L. Methylene blue-encapsulated phosphonate-terminated silica nanoparticles for simultaneous *in vivo* imaging and photodynamic therapy. Biomaterials 2009; 30(29): 5601-9.
[http://dx.doi.org/10.1016/j.biomaterials.2009.06.030] [PMID: 19595455]

[215]   Królicki L, Bruchertseifer F, Kunikowska J, *et al.* Safety and efficacy of targeted alpha therapy with [213]Bi-DOTA-substance P in recurrent glioblastoma. Eur J Nucl Med Mol Imaging 2019; 46(3): 614-22.
[http://dx.doi.org/10.1007/s00259-018-4225-7] [PMID: 30498897]

SUBJECT INDEX

A

B

K

Kainic acid 78

L

Lennox-Gastaut Syndrome 39
Lesions 79, 116, 120, 121, 129, 126, 135
  cerebral 120
  high-grade 129
  intracerebral 126
  neoplastic 121, 126
  nonneoplastic 121
  pathological 79
Lethal genetic neurodegenerative disease 76
Leukopenia 43
Ligand functionalization 133
Lipolysis 48
  beta-adrenergic receptors stimulate 48
Lipooligosaccharides 73
Lyme disease 72
Lymphangiogenesis progress 113
Lymphocytes 67, 72, 73

M

Macrocyclic chelating ligand 131
Magnetic resonance imaging (MRI) 75, 109,
    110, 111, 115, 118, 119, 123, 124, 125,
    127, 128, 129, 133, 135
Malabsorption 40
MAPK activation signalling pathway 70
MAP kinase 70
Mechanisms 1, 3, 10, 22, 23, 37, 41, 42, 44,
    48, 60, 67, 109, 120, 122, 130
  autoregulatory 3
  defence 60
  genetic 109, 111
  hybridization 130
  hyperexcitability 67
  pathogenetic 23
Medications 36, 40, 44, 69, 91
  anticonvulsant 69
  anti-obesity 40
  antipsychotic 44, 91
Medulloblastomas 110
Meningitis 60, 61, 62, 63
  bacterial 61, 62
  herpes 61

Meningococcal vaccines 63
Mesenchymal stem cell 79
Metabolic 38, 45, 49, 124
  homeostasis 45
  syndrome 38, 49
Metabolism 12, 41, 43, 48, 113, 128, 139
  fatty acid 41
  hepatic 113
  lipid 48
  synthesis functions 128
  targeting tumor 139
Migraine 37, 38, 40, 46, 47, 48, 49, 50
  familial hemiplegic 49
  prophylaxis 38, 40, 47, 48, 49, 50
Mitochondria 77, 78, 80
  -directed therapies 77
  dysfunction 78
  dynamics modulators 80
Monophosphate-activated protein kinase 69
Motor neuron disease (MND) 4
Multifunctional drug delivery systems 110
Muscarinic cholinergic receptors 49
Muscle atrophy, progressive 1
Mycoplasma pneumonia 73
Myostatin inhibitors 10, 20, 21

N

Nanosized contrast agents (NCAs) 118
Nausea 94, 96
Necrosis 109, 111, 121, 123, 126, 127, 139
  radiation 121, 123
Negative inspiratory force (NIF) 75
Neoangiogenesis 114
Neoplasms 13, 119
  intracranial 119
Neovascularization 114
Nerve damage 67, 72
  facial 72
Nerve injury 67, 68
  central 67, 68
  peripheral 67, 68
Nervous system 60, 61, 67, 72, 80
  peripheral 61, 72
  sympathetic 45
Nervous system disorders 60, 80
  respective 80
  treating 60

T

Targeting 9, 23, 65, 76, 110, 114, 115, 119, 131, 132, 133, 136, 138, 139
  autoimmune disease 76
  DNA 65
  ligands 138
  SMN protein 9
Target protein 111
Techniques 111, 115, 116
  mediated imaging 116
  mediated molecular imaging 116
  radiological 115
  radiological imaging 111
Therapy 1, 10, 11, 16, 17, 19, 97, 98, 111, 112, 113, 114, 131, 132, 133, 134, 135, 137, 138, 139
  adjunctive 19
  adjuvant temozolomide 113
  dopaminergic agonist 98
  gene-based SMA 17
  gene replacement 17
  gene transfer 16
  image-guided radiation 135
  oestrogen-replacement 98
  photodynamic 137
  radionuclidic 138
  targeted 60, 138
  targeted alpha 139
  tumor-activated prodrug 133
Thermal hyperalgesia 70
Thrombocytopenia 23
Thyroid hormone 40
Tissues 15, 17, 62, 77, 79, 92, 111, 113, 118
  cerebral 77
  embryonic striatal 79
  live tumor 118
  necrotic 118
  non-neuronal 15
Tobramycin 19
Transferrin receptors 119
Transgene translation 16
Translation 11, 23
  modulating SMN protein 11
Transmission electron microscopy 134
Transsphenoidal surgery (TS) 97
Treatment 14, 17, 37, 42, 43, 53
  antipsychotic 42, 43
  antipsychotic drug 53
  disease-modifying 14

dopaminergic 42
lifelong intrathecal 17
nusinersen 14
prophylactic 37
Tumor 111, 112, 113, 117, 118, 119, 120, 121, 123, 127, 128, 129, 130, 133, 134, 137, 138
  angiogenesis 113, 130
  diagnosis 133
  hypoxia 128
  invasiveness 119
  malignancy 117, 127
  margins 120
  necrosis 111, 118
  prognosis 128, 134
  therapy 138
  tissue 112, 121, 123, 129, 137
Tumor cell 139
  death 139
  metabolism 139

U

Upconversion luminescence (UCL) 134

V

Valproic acid (VPA) 11, 14, 36, 37, 38, 40, 64, 65, 70
Vascular endothelial growth factor (VEGF) 79, 111, 112, 113, 118
  receptor 118
Vectors 16, 65, 70
  adeno-associated virus 65
  enkephalin-expressing 70
Voltage-gated 37, 65
  Ca channel modulator 37
  potassium channel 65
  sodium channel inactivation 37

W

Weight gain 35, 36, 37, 38, 39, 40, 41, 42, 43, 44, 45, 46, 47, 48, 49, 50, 53
  antipsychotics cause 44
  drug-induced 36, 53
Weight-neutral drugs 37
Werdnig-Hoffmann disease 5